# Ligamentous Articular Strain

## Osteopathic Manipulative Techniques for the Body

# Ligamentous Articular Strain

## Osteopathic Manipulative Techniques for the Body

Conrad A. Speece, D.O. and William Thomas Crow, D.O.
Illustrated by Steven L. Simmons, D.O.

EASTLAND PRESS • SEATTLE

Published by Eastland Press, Incorporated
P.O. Box 99749, Seattle, WA 98199 USA
All rights reserved.

International Standard Book Number:  0-939616-31-9
Library of Congress Catalog Card Number:  98-74969
Printed in the Republic of Korea

2  4  6  8  10  9  7  5  3  1


Book design by Gordon Frazier
Cover design by Lilian Lai Bensky
Cover illustration from *On the Structure of the Human Body* (1543) by Andreas Vesalius

# Table of Contents

# *Preface*

William Garner Sutherland, D.O., taught many ways of addressing clinical problems in the practice of Osteopathy. In all views, he emphasized the fact that the living human body is one physiological organism. Study groups, such as the Dallas Osteopathic Study Group, are making these teachings available to the profession today. This book introduces the reader to valuable ways of using ligamentous articular balance and myofascial release methods. Dr. Sutherland taught that the goal of an Osteopathic treatment is to effect a more efficient interchange among all the fluids of the body at all interfaces.

In the practice of Osteopathy, the physician keeps the basic facts of anatomy and physiology in mind, together with the particular problems that his patients bring him. He has to find the problem, understand it, and plan a program of treatment for solving it. The plan of treatment may vary, but the result should be normal action. The principles of ligamentous articular strain and of myofascial release provide valuable information for use in practice. This book has much useful knowledge for Osteopathic practice.

*Anne L. Wales, D.O., D.Sc. (hon.)*
*North Attleboro, MA*

# CHAPTER ONE

# Introduction

The goals of this book are: (1) To provide the serious practitioner and student of osteopathy with the opportunity to learn manipulative techniques for treating various parts of the body based on the work of Andrew Taylor Still, M.D., and William G. Sutherland, D.O., and (2) To provide a methodology for considering the human body as a whole, rather than just the sum of its parts

In order to gain the most from this text, you need to have a deep understanding of the interactions among the parts of the body, including the bones, and of the body's mechanisms for maintaining homeostasis. These are needed to understand the treatment approach taught in this book and to effectively use the techniques, resulting in dramatic treatments.

In addition, this book will aid you in developing a unique style for treating patients. An artist develops his or her own style after long years of studying the works and techniques of masters. The Dallas Osteopathic Study Group has been our studio, and Rollin Becker, D.O., Alan Becker, D.O., Herb Miller, D.O., Robert Fulford, D.O., and many other "grand masters" have coached us through the years. We have included in this book some of their techniques as well as those developed by members of the Dallas Osteopathic Study Group.

All of the techniques included here were developed over the thirty-plus years that the Dallas Osteopathic Study Group has been studying osteopathic manipulative treatment techniques. They are a distillation of the hundreds of techniques that have been developed by members of the Dallas Osteopathic Study Group or brought into the Dallas Osteopathic Study Group from outside conferences. Many of the techniques that are not included were eliminated because, though effective, they were ergonomic nightmares. In order to enjoy a long and productive career, the practitioner needs to conserve energy and not stress or strain his or her own body by using poor body mechanics while treating patients.

Initially, the focus of the Dallas Osteopathic Study Group was on cranial osteopathy. Then, in 1982, the study group began an extensive study of the indirect and direct methods of osteopathic manipulative treatment set forth in a 1949 article by H.A. Lippincott,[1] which will be discussed in greater detail in Chapter 2. Most of the indirect techniques found in Lippincott's article are now called *ligamentous articular strain techniques* while several of them also form the basis of *myofascial release techniques.*

Over the years, the Dallas Osteopathic Study Group and its individual members found that there were ways to improve some of the earlier techniques. The main difference between the original ligamentous articular strain techniques found in the Lippincott article and the new techniques described here is that the original techniques have been modified to be more ergonomically efficient and to require little or no patient cooperation. This was done because asking for patient cooperation often leads to the patient tensing up while trying to comply with the request, which tends to interfere with the treatment.

A. T. Still concentrated on teaching the philosophy of osteopathy because he did not want to lock the minds of future osteopaths into his techniques.[2] By definition, a technique is a procedure that utilizes a position, method, and activating force. Thus, a technique is just another word for grip. Dr. Still's feeling was that if a practitioner understood and adhered to the philosophy of osteopathy, that is, an understanding of the mechanisms of the body and of the principles of osteopathy, that individual could develop his or her own techniques.[3]

We have attempted to provide you here with the benefits of the Dallas Osteopathic Study Group's search since 1963 for easier, more user-friendly, and effective techniques that treat the body from the head down and that apply Dr. Still's principles. To that end, the book is divided into three sections. Section I traces the roots of the techniques and provides the general principles required to perform them, covering joint physiology, fluid dynamics, the role of the fascia, and the concept of vectors of injury. Section II sets forth detailed techniques for treating the various areas of the body, except for the cranium. Section III ties the body together as a functional unit.

Treatment of the cranium is not covered in this book, as those techniques have been well described in other texts. A good reference book for these techniques is *Osteopathy in the Cranial Field* by Harold I. Magoun, D.O.[4]

The operating principle that has guided both the Dallas Osteopathic Study Group and this book is best articulated by Rollin Becker, D.O.:

> When you learn to listen to the body physiology of the patient, you may not look like you are doing anything outwardly, but you're working hard; it's hard work to listen for any length of time. But you can learn to do it, and you have the rest of your practice life. Still and Sutherland did it, I don't know why you can't. Dr. Still and Dr. Sutherland were students. They spent their entire lives studying the science of osteopathy, and one of the fundamental things they learned was that there is no time in which you can ever quit learning about the science of osteopathy. They consented to be used by the fundamental laws that are within each body physiology. They learned to know and use the rules of health as they apply within us, and it is these rules that are sought in the restoration to health for any dysfunction, disease, or trauma for which the patient is seeking service. Dr. Still and Dr. Sutherland studied every single mechanism within the body physiology as it applied to a given patient, and they were taught by each individual case the appropriate diagnostic and treatment program. They were taught by that which the body itself was trying to do.

What is new in the science of osteopathy? The answer is simple: the next patient who walks in the office, the one who has been everywhere and tried everything. The body physiology is the teacher and the physician is the student. The mechanism of body physiology offers many doors for experimentation to promote better health. You, as the physician-student, create techniques based on understanding the mechanism, visualizing what you think should be for that area, and then developing techniques as you understand the mechanism for each individual case and each individual patient. In other words, you are allowed lots of room for experimentation, as long as you obey the laws of the science of osteopathy. You get results in proportion to your knowledge and your developing sense of touch. We, as students of body physiology, as physicians, can use and be used by the body physiology of the patient in the care of each individual patient. The future is very bright for those who choose to study and use the works of Dr. Still and Dr. Sutherland. Thank you.[5]

---

[1] Lippincott HA. "The Osteopathic Technique of Wm. G. Sutherland, D.O." in *1949 Yearbook of the Academy of Applied Osteopathy*. Reprint, Indianapolis, IN: American Academy of Osteopathy.

[2] Still AT. *Osteopathy: Research and Practice.* Kirksville, MO: The Journal Printing Company, 1910: 41.

[3] Ibid., 53.

[4] Magoun HI. *Osteopathy in the Cranial Field,* 3rd ed. Indianapolis, IN: The Cranial Academy, 1976.

[5] Ibid., 8–9.

# SECTION I

# Historical Background and Principles

# CHAPTER TWO

# History

# Background

As previously noted, the initial focus of the Dallas Osteopathic Study Group (DOSG) was on cranial osteopathy. Then, in 1982, the study group shifted its focus from techniques for treating the head to techniques for treating the whole body. The DOSG felt it would begin its search for effective techniques by investigating the approaches used by its predecessors. This came about due to the efforts of two of our most influential and well-respected members, now deceased, Neil Pruzzo, D.O. and Rollin Becker, D.O. Dr. Pruzzo was looking for a topic for the 1984 Cranial Academy Conference which was to be held in Fort Worth, Texas. Dr. Becker suggested that the DOSG present a course on Ligamentous Articular Strain, as it had not been taught since 1947. Dr. Becker had been in attendance at the 1947 presentation and had used those techniques ever since, so he was able to guide the members in their study and eventual mastery. Accordingly, the DOSG began an extensive study of the indirect and direct methods of osteopathic manipulative treatment (OMT) found in the 1949 article by H.A. Lippincott[1] that recorded Dr. Sutherland's 1947 presentation to his study group, and was his only lecture on ligamentous articular strain techniques.

In the late 1980s, while attending a course on ligamentous articular strain given by the DOSG, Brian Knight, D.O., related that several years previously he was treating a very elderly gentleman with the techniques outlined in this text. The patient expressed delight at finding someone who treated like Dr. A. T. Still. He said that as a young man, Dr. Still treated him and that Still had used those very techniques.[2]

This information piqued the interest of the members of the study group as to the history of the techniques taught by W. G. Sutherland, D.O., and the techniques taught by Dr. Still.

In addition, the study group wanted to know whether those techniques were used to treat both the head as well as the rest of the body. The search was conducted by talking to people who knew Sutherland, or had a historical connection to Still, and by reviewing the early literature.

# First-Hand Interviews

In March, 1995, Brooks Walker, D.O., who was then in his mid-80s, was questioned at the A.A.O. Convocation in Nashville, Tennessee. As Dr. Walker had studied with Sutherland, and his mother had graduated in the 1902 class and studied directly with A.T. Still, he was in a good position to know whether or not some of the techniques taught by Sutherland had come from Still. In fact, while Dr. Walker was studying with Dr. Sutherland in the

1940s, he had questioned his mother about whether Dr. Still had treated the head. She confirmed that he had.

People like Alan Becker, D.O., who personally studied with Sutherland and whose father had studied with Still, were also questioned. They confirmed that A.T. Still had indeed treated the head as well as the rest of the body. Sutherland went on to say that Still's problem was that he was so involved with running the school that he had founded in Kirksville that he did not have time to expand on the motion of the individual bones of the cranium. Thus, he told Sutherland to "dig on."[3]

# W. G. Sutherland

William G. Sutherland, D.O., who first presented osteopathy in the cranial field in the late 1930s, became frustrated that it was being presented separately from osteopathy of the body. As a result, he taught a course in 1947 to reinforce the connection between osteopathy of the head and of the body, and to show what Still had taught about the rest of the body.[4] As noted above, this course formed the basis of the 1949 article written by H.A. Lippincott, D.O., in which he wrote:

> At the time that Dr. Sutherland received his osteopathic training at Kirskville, Dr. Andrew Taylor Still was carefully supervising all the instruction given at the college. The principles that were taught had to conform exactly to his concept. Dr. Sutherland made good use of every opportunity to learn and understand them and has adhered closely in his thinking and practice to Dr. Still's principles throughout his professional career. In consequence, the technique which he presented to us is a reflection of the clear vision of our founder.[5]

At the beginning of this course, Dr. Sutherland exploded when asked by his followers for more cranial methods.[6] He told them that this was "Osteopathy" and nothing more. He went on to say that they were as bad as the rest of the profession, except that they were decapitating the body and throwing it away, while the rest of the profession was throwing away the head. At this session, which apparently lasted for a few weeks, he did not say anything about the cranium, just the rest of the body.

In his transcribed lectures, W. G. Sutherland reflected on his training and how by utilizing the principles of osteopathy, he had learned to treat problems that surgeons treated with scalpels. In *Teachings in the Science of Osteopathy*, Sutherland stated:

> From the study of the ligamentous articular mechanism of the pelvis, I learned enough so that I could compete with the needle and with the methods of ambulant proctology in my own profession. Thinking

osteopathy with Dr. Still and with this view of anatomy, I developed several methods I called lap techniques.[7]

Also, he made the point that certain structures of the body act as ligaments and could be treated the same way that the ligaments are treated.

> The leg is a membranous articular mechanism. So is the forearm. There is the tibiofibular interosseus membrane and the radioulnar membrane. You can use these membranes as you use ligaments to realign the relations between the bones. This is because they function like ligaments in the regional mechanisms.[8]

In addition, before explaining a treatment performed by A. T. Still, Sutherland emphasized the importance of looking at distal effects of an injury and its effect on the fascia, which can react like ligamentous structures. During this course, Sutherland related the following:

> Dr. Still gave me a lesson one day along with the rest of our class. A member of our class had stepped on a rusty nail. All the appropriate surgical management and cleansing had been used, but it would not heal. It began to look an angry red, so we called in the Old Doctor. He said, 'You damn fools!' and we were. We had not stopped to consider that when the patient stepped on that nail he drew his leg up away from it. The lasting problem was not the nail or the original wound; it was what occurred in the sudden jerk of the patient that caused a membranous strain between the fibula and the tibia.[9]

Sutherland wrote the following about how Still would treat the membranous strain (i.e., the fascia):

> Technic: In all spinal technic it is my custom to have the patient exercise his own natural forces rather than the application of mine. There are no thrusts, no jerks nor the application of another or distal end of the anatomy as a lever. *The principle is that used and taught by Dr. Still, namely, exaggeration of the lesion to the degree of release and then allowing the ligaments to draw the articulations back into normal relationship.* This same method is applied in sacroiliac technic.[10]

Sutherland's student H. A. Lippincott, D.O., elaborated on this:

> Since it is the ligaments that are primarily involved in the maintenance of the lesion it is they, not muscular leverage, that are used as the main agency for reduction. The articulation is carried in the direction of the lesion position as far as is necessary to cause tension of the weakened elements of the ligamentous structure to be equal to or slight in excess of the tension of those that are not strained. This is the point of balanced tension. Forcing the articulation back and away from the direction of lesion strains the ligaments that are normal and unopposed, and if it is done with thrust or jerks there is a definite possibility of separat-

ing fibers of ligaments from their bony attachments. When the tension is properly balanced the respiratory or muscular cooperation of the patient is employed to overcome the resistance of the defense mechanism of the body to the release of the lesion.[11]

Sutherland is best remembered for his application of osteopathic techniques for the cranium and sacrum. However, it is clear that he had learned from Dr. Still techniques for treating the whole body, and was only expounding more on an area that was receiving insufficient attention at that time, that is, the motion of the individual bones in the cranium. This is why Sutherland, later in his life, held that he had just pulled back a veil so that others could see more clearly.

# A. T. Still

Still spent a good number of years in the late 19th century trying out a number of different methods of treatment. When he finally started the first osteopathic college in 1892, he taught what used to be called *traction methods*, which are known today as *indirect methods*.[12] Most of these methods later became known as ligamentous articular strain techniques, while several of them also formed the basis of myofascial release techniques. These methods were all but replaced in the early 20th century by direct methods, which are primarily *high velocity–low amplitude*, familiarly known as "crunching." This does not mean, however, that A.T. Still did not himself use some form of high velocity–low amplitude technique, since he was also known as the "lightning bonesetter."[13]

While ligamentous articular strain techniques may not be the only techniques used by Drs. Still and Sutherland, they are the ones which both of them described. For example, Dr. Still wrote:

> Without going into detail further, I will say that all dislocations, partial or complete, can be adjusted by this rule: First loosen the dislocated end from other tissues, then gently bring it back to its original place.[14]

And there is also this about treating the cervical spine:

> Draw your patient about six inches beyond the end of the table, bring pressure to bear upon the head down toward the body in order that the muscles of the neck can become loosened or shortened. Thus, you will see that your work is to readjust the muscles and permit the articulations to return to normal.[15]

Carl Phillip McConnell, D.O., M.D., who had been treated by Still and was on the faculty at the American School of Osteopathy, described Still's treatment technique in his book, *The Practice of Osteopathy*:

Disengage the articular points that have become locked. Reduce the dis-location by retracing the path along which the parts were dislocated. One can readily see that a dislocated ball and socket joint could be reduced only by the dislocated bone retracing the path through which it left its socket as the capsular ligament would at once prevent its returning to the socket by any path other than that taken when dislocated. This applies to all dislocations to a greater or lesser extent.[16]

This is one of the earliest writings about Still's technique from a source other than Still himself.

Still tried to share with his audience his notions concerning appropriate treatments. However, there is little written about techniques that Still used, nor did he write very much about specific techniques. In *The Philosophy of Osteopathy* he explained why:

It is my object in this work to teach principles as I understand them, and not rules. I do not instruct the student to push or pull a certain bone, nerve or muscle for a certain disease, but by a knowledge of the normal and abnormal, I hope to give a specific knowledge for all disease.[17]

Keep a living picture before your mind all the time, so you can see all joints, ligaments, muscles, glands, arteries, veins, lymphatics, fascia superficial and deep, all organs, how they are fed, what they must do, and why they are expected to do a part, and what would follow in case that part was not done well and on time. Keep your minds full of pictures of the normal body all the time, while treating the afflicted.[18]

In *Osteopathy: Research and Practice* Still wrote:

The mechanical principles upon which osteopathy is based are as old as the universe.[19]

As an educated engineer of five years' schooling I began to look at the human framework as a machine and examined all its parts to see if I could find any variation from the truly normal among its journals, belts, pulleys, and escape pipes . . . When all parts of the human body are in line we have health. When they are not the effect is disease. When the parts are readjusted disease gives place to health.[20]

In teaching ligamentous articular strain to students we often tell them that the dysfunctional part of the body feels "hard." This concept of "hard" comes from various sources in the literature. Edward Goetz, D.O., in *A Manual of Osteopathy with the Application of Physical Culture, Baths and Diet*, discussed the "rules of osteopathy." Here is rule number seven:

The idea of manipulation of the muscles is to soften them to restore the circulation and to relieve the pressure on nerves impinged upon the contracture or hardening of the muscles, hence sufficient time must be given to accomplish this.[21]

In helping the "hard part" of the body soften, you must try to take the body into the position of ease by doing what Dr. Still wrote:

> A normal image of the form and function of all parts of the body must be seen by the mind's eye or our work will condemn us.[22]

This hardness is caused by lack of fluid (blood, interstitial fluid) flowing through an area of dysfunction. An example of this can be found in the following advice given by Dr. Still:

> ... the thigh bone having openings, or doors, to receive arterial blood at the upper end. A partial or complete dislocation of the head of the femur from the socket would naturally shut off the blood supply. A dislocation of the femur produces a twist of the muscle about the neck of the bone, including the muscles and membranes that are stretched and producing a pressure sufficient to shut off the nerve and blood supply to this bone. Then we have inflammatory rheumatism. We are in possession of the knowledge to the cause that has produced this abnormality. Allow yourself to think of the nerve and blood supply to the acetabula, innominate, sacrum and spine from the socket to the brain.[23]

Elsewhere, Dr. Still emphasized the need to work with the connective tissues of the body, the fascia, muscles and ligaments:

> Previous to readjusting any bone in the body, it matters not from which one it is or how far it has been forced from its socket, you must first loosen it at its attachments at its articulating end, always bearing in mind that when a bone has left its proper articulation the surrounding muscles and ligaments are irritated and keep up a continual contracture.[24]

Still used these principles when treating, for example, the hip:

> Without going into further detail I will say that all dislocations, partial or complete, can be adjusted by this rule: First loosen the dislocated end from other tissues, then gently bring it back to its original place.
> A fixed point, a lever, a twist, or a screw power, can be and are used by all operators. It is not a matter of imitation but the bringing the bone from the abnormal to the normal.[25]

Another description of the techniques used in the early days of Osteopathy is given in the writings of Edythe Ashmore, D.O., who was a student of Still's and a professor of Osteopathic Mechanics at the American School of Osteopathy. In her 1915 book *Osteopathic Mechanics*, she describes osteopathic techniques:

> General Rules—The articulating surfaces must retrace the path they took in their displacement. It has been well said that it requires but a

little force at exactly the right angle to produce a lesion, and conversely that a little force applied in exactly the right direction will reduce a subluxation. There are two methods commonly employed by osteopaths in the correction of lesions, the older of which is the traction method, the later the direct method or thrust.[26]

In a footnote, she wrote:

The term 'direct' is preferred for the reason that the imitators of osteopathy have given to the word 'thrust' an objectionable meaning of harshness.[27]

As noted previously, the older method is now known as ligamentous articular strain techniques, while the newer methods refer to high velocity–low amplitude techniques. Of the former, she wrote:

Those who employ the traction method secure the relaxation of the tissues about the articulation by what has been termed exaggeration of the lesion, a motion in the direction of the forcible movement which produced the lesion, as if its purpose were to increase the deformity. C.P. McConnell states that this disengages the tissues that are holding the parts in the abnormal position. The exaggeration is held, traction made upon the joint, replacement initiated and then completed by reversal of the forces.[28]

Dr. Ashmore went on to say that the indirect methods were more difficult than the direct methods and, therefore, should not be used in the instruction of students. While we would have to agree that ligamentous articular strain may be somewhat harder to learn than some of the more common osteopathic techniques, it has been done successfully by the DOSG and at several Osteopathic schools.

It is true that many modern patients are fond of the high velocity–low amplitude techniques, in part because of the resulting "pop" from the patient's joint. However, the pop itself does not improve the patient's condition, and high velocity–low amplitude techniques are not necessarily the best methods of treatment for a given patient. This subject was addressed by Dr. Still:

One man advises to pull out a bone to attempt to set until they pop. That popping is no criterion to go by. Bones do not always pop when they go back into their proper place, nor does it mean they are properly adjusted when they do pop. If you pull your finger you will hear a sudden noise. The sudden and forcible separation of the ends of the bones that form the joint causes a vacuum and the air entering from about the joint to fill the vacuum causes the explosive noise.[29]

# Summary

The Dallas Osteopathic Study Group's strong commitment to A.T. Still's principles was the basis for its intense interest in finding out if Sutherland learned ligamentous articular strain techniques from Dr. Still himself. After all, the general principles taught by A. T. Still were to disengage, exaggerate, and balance. As he emphasized over and over, if you learn the principles of osteopathy, you can apply them to any part of the body.

The ligamentous articular strain techniques are not new, and they are not the only method that can be used to treat a patient. However, the techniques have been used successfully for over a century. Our feeling is that, even if ligamentous articular strain was not taught to Sutherland by Still, it does not diminish its importance in the armamentarium of the osteopathic physician. As Dr. Still so eloquently explained:

> I want to make it plain that there are many ways of adjusting bones. And when one operator does not use the same method as another, it does not show criminal ignorance, but simply getting of results in a different manner. . . . The choice of methods is a matter to be decided by each operator and depends on his own skill and judgement. . . . It is not a matter of imitation and doing just as some successful operator does, but bringing of the bone from the abnormal to the normal.[30]

---

1  Lippincott HA. "The Osteopathic Techniques of Wm. G. Sutherland, D.O." in 1949 Yearbook of the Academy of Applied Osteopathy. Reprint, Indianapolis, IN: American Academy of Osteopathy.

2  Personal communication with authors.

3  Personal communication from Alan Becker to Conrad Speece, AAO Convocation, Nashville, 1997.

4  Personal communication from John Fox  to W. T. Crow.

5  Lippincott, "Osteopathic Techniques of Sutherland," 1.

6  The story was handed down by word of mouth from Rollin and Alan Becker and confirmed by John Fox, all of whom studied under Sutherland and were present at the 1947 conference.

7  Sutherland WG. *Teachings in the Science of Osteopathy*, ed. Anne Wales, D.O. Portland, OR: Rudra Press, 1990: 187.

8  Ibid., 188.

9  Ibid.

10  Ibid., 94.

11  Lippincott, "Osteopathic Techniques of Sutherland," 1.

12  Ashmore EF. *Osteopathic Mechanics: A Textbook.* Kirksville, MO: The Journal Printing Company, 1915: 72.

13  Still AT. *Autobiography of A. T. Still : With a History of the Discovery of and Development of the Science of Osteopathy,* rev. ed. Kirksville, MO: The Journal Printing Company, 1908.

14  Still AT. *Osteopathy: Research and Practice.* Kirksville, MO: The Journal Printing Company, 1910: 53.

15  Ibid., 265–66.

16  McConnell CP. *Practice of Osteopathy.* Kirksville, MO: Journal Printing Company, 1906: 58.

17  Still AT. *Philosophy of Osteopathy.* Kirksville, MO: The Journal Printing Company, 1899: 4.

18  Ibid., 13.

19  Still, *Osteopathy: Research and Practice,* vi.

20  Ibid., vii.

21  Goetz E. *A Manual of Osteopathy with the Application of Physical Culture, Baths and Diet.* Cincinnati, OH: Nature's Cure Publishing, 1905: 13.

22  Still, *Osteopathy: Research and Practice,* 41.

23  Ibid., 43.

24  Ibid., 52–53.

25  Ibid., 55.

26  Ashmore, *Osteopathic Mechanics,* 72.

27  Ibid., 72.

28  Ibid.

29  Still, *Osteopathy: Research and Practice,* 52.

30  Ibid., 55.

# CHAPTER THREE

# The Scientific Basis and Principles Underlying Ligamentous Articular Release

Although the title of this book is *Ligamentous Articular Strain*, ligaments are not the only structures that are addressed. Using modern terminology, many of these techniques could be considered as examples of myofascial release. Yet we chose the title *Ligamentous Articular Strain* because we believe these techniques are based on the original principles used by Dr. Sutherland and Dr. Still before classifications like myofascial release were introduced. To our study group, this is osteopathy as it was originally taught. In this chapter, we will explore the scientific basis and principles underlying these methods.

# Ligamentous Articular Strains

When treating a patient with dysfunctions, keep a mental image of the normal anatomy and function as well as of the embryology. Remember that we start from one cell and divide into two cells, four cells, and so forth. In the early stages of the embryo, the only circulatory system that is needed is the rhythmic motion of the interstitial fluid. When the embryo becomes too large to absorb or diffuse all of it as nutrients and waste products through its surface, it develops a cardiovascular system to carry the nutrition to the far reaches of its body and to carry the waste products away. The cardiovascular system coupled with the rhythmic motion of the interstitial fluid bathes equally every cell of the fetus. Later, when the need for maintenance of the shape and form arises, the skeletal system develops. This eventually is followed by the need to bear weight, so the skeletal system develops to allow for the normal involuntary as well as voluntary motions of the body. Never lose sight of the fact that form and function are totally interrelated, and that function dictates form.

The term *ligamentous articular strain* most accurately describes the somatic dysfunction that occurs in the ligamentous structures that surround a joint. The tension in all of the ligaments of a normal joint is balanced and is used to center adjacent bones in their articular grooves and spaces. This suspension system keeps the bones from being jammed too close together, pulled too far apart, shifted from one side to the other, twisted, or bent sideways. When an injury occurs, one bone in the joint becomes jammed beyond this physiologic position, and some, if not all, of the ligaments become strained. Of the pair of opposing ligaments, the more lax ligament is usually the more strained ligament, while the tighter ligament is more normal.[1]

The goal of treatment is to balance the tension in both ligaments and maintain that equal tension until the body recenters the bones by tightening the lax ligament. Once the joint is returned to its normal physiologic position, the ligaments can begin a three-month healing process, which is the time it takes for connective tissue to regenerate.[2] If the joint is not restrained during this process, further treatment of this joint is not required.

H. A. Lippincott, D.O., describes ligamentous articular strain as follows:

> Osteopathic lesions are strains of the tissues of the body. When they involve joints, it is the ligaments that are primarily affected so the term "ligamentous articular strain" is the one preferred by Dr. Sutherland. The ligaments of a joint are normally on a balanced, reciprocal tension and seldom if ever are they completely relaxed throughout the normal range of movement. When the motion is carried beyond that range, the tension is unbalanced and the elements of the ligamentous structure that limit motion in that direction are strained and weakened. The lesion is maintained by the overbalance of the reciprocal tension by the elements that have not been strained. This locks the articular mechanism or prevents its free and normal movement. The unbalanced tension causes the bones to assume a position that is nearer that in which the strain was produced than would be the case if the tension were normal, and the weakened part of the ligaments permits motion in the direction of the lesion in excess of normal. The range of movement in the opposite direction is limited by the more firm and unopposed tension of the elements which had not been strained.[3]

It should be noted that a significant number of the treatment techniques in this book deal with muscles, tendons, and fascia. Strains in these structures are more correctly referred to as *myofascial strains*, and the methods used to correct them as *myofascial release.*

# Principles of Corrective Technique

Once an area of dysfunction has been located, compress or decompress the joint or fascial plane to disengage the injury so that the displaced bone can be moved. (This is similar to pushing in the clutch on a car to shift gears.) Then carry the injured part in the direction of least resistance, returning it to the original position to which it was forced during the injury. Carrying the injury the way it wants to go is an *indirect method* of treatment and is also one that follows the direction of the somatic dysfunction. Remember that just after the initial injury, the injured part sprang back toward a normal position but was caught in limbo—part way between the position of the injury and the normal functional position. So, when correcting the injury, you must carry the injured part back to the exact position of injury and maintain that position until the body rebalances all the connective tissue surrounding the dysfunction, and draws the part back to its normal functional physiologic position. This can be done using a direct technique, an indirect technique, or a combination of indirect and direct methods.

*Ligamentous articular release* and *myofascial release* are probably best thought of as activating forces. It is the act of disengagement, exaggeration, and balance that makes the techniques work. These are the three basic components to remember when utilizing ligamentous articular strain techniques: disengage, exaggerate, and balance.

1. Disengage: Compress or decompress the joint or fascial plane, increasing the pressure or traction until you are able to move the injured part.

2. Exaggerate: Carry the injured part back to the original position of injury by, for example, rotating, flexing, "side-bending," or "side-shifting" until the balance point or still point is found. For example, if the right ankle is slightly inverted, you exaggerate the position of the ankle by taking it into a more inverted position, which is how the injury occurred originally.

3. Balance: Maintain the area of dysfunction in the position of injury, that is, the balance point or still point, until a release occurs. The bone will move slightly farther in the direction of exaggeration. It then will move back to its normal functional position as the *cranial rhythmic impulse* or *tide* returns through the tissues that were injured. Once the correction has occurred, the injured ligaments will start their three-month healing process.

# Nomenclature

The descriptions of the techniques used in the next section include the position of the patient, the method utilized, and type of release that occurs. The positions used in this text are:

- Supine: Patient is lying on his or her back.

- Prone: Patient is lying on his or her stomach.

- Lateral recumbent: Patient is lying on his or her side.

The methods describe the action taken to set up the technique. The methods used in this text are:

- Indirect: Carrying the injured part in the direction that caused the injury.

- Direct: Carrying the injured part toward its normal position.

- Combined: Initially using the indirect method, and as the technique is completed, the movements becomes direct.

The treatment is complete when a release occurs. The types of release referred to in this text are:

- Ligamentous articular release: Refers to treatments that are applied to ligaments and articular structures.

- Myofascial release: Refers to treatments that are applied to muscles, tendons, or fascia.

Examples include *lateral recumbent–indirect–ligamentous articular release* for the shoulder or *supine–direct–myofascial release* for the pelvic diaphragm. Diagnosis is based upon palpation of the appropriate structures to feel for "strains" or restricted motion. In many instances, diagnosis and treatment occur simultaneously because the treatment position is determined by the motion preferences that are felt in the tissues. It is based upon finding areas of restriction in the spine and treating those areas by disengaging the facets and balancing the tissue tension until a release is felt.

The principle is similar in the sacrum, which can have many types of dysfunction occurring around multiple axes of motion. After the disengagement, the exaggeration and balance follow the direction dictated by the sacrum. As noted above, diagnosis and treatment often occur at the same time. It is important to point out that a nonphysiologic dysfunction of the sacrum, often referred to as an "innominate," such as an innominate shear, should probably be checked for and corrected first.

Treatment order is discussed more in the latter chapters of the book. One thing that should be evident is that it takes practice to be able to feel dysfunctions in body structures. The more you practice, the more you will be able to quickly feel when a myofascial structure is strained or a joint is restricted.

Most of the techniques covered in this text are indirect, as these methods are usually less painful and traumatic for the patient. When direct methods are used, they are nonthrusting movements and involve the use of balanced, steady pressure toward relocating the bone to its normal physiologic position.

The principles of corrective techniques are described by Lippincott as follows:

> Since it is the ligaments that are primarily involved in the maintenance of the lesion, it is they, not muscular leverage, that are used as the main agency for reduction. The articulation is carried in the direction of the lesion, exaggerating the lesion position as far as is necessary to cause the tension of the weakened elements of the ligamentous structure to be equal to or slightly in excess of the tension of those that were not strained. This is the point of balanced tension. Forcing the joint to move beyond that point adds to the strain which is already present. Forcing the articulation back and away from the direction of lesion strains the ligaments that are normal and unopposed, and if it is done with thrusts or jerks there is a definite possibility of separating fibers of the ligaments from their bony attachments.[4]

# Fluid Dynamics

As noted previously, in the embryo, the movement of the interstitial fluid precedes temporally the development of the cardiovascular system. We feel that this motion represents the equivalent of the cranial rhythmic impulse in the embryo. An additional goal of the treatments is to restore function to the dysfunctional areas that lack this fluid motion.[5] When this has been accomplished, the motion of the cranial rhythmic impulse returns to the treated tissues.

The cranial rhythmic impulse was commonly called the *tide* by Dr. Sutherland because of its rhythmic ebb and flow. Although this rhythmic motion includes "cranial" as part of its name, it is present and can be felt throughout the entire body. This rhythmic motion of the interstitial fluid bathes all the cells so that the nutrients are carried from the capillaries to the cells and the waste products are carried from the cells to the capillaries. This tide ebbs and flows like the tides and waves of the ocean.

At a Dallas Osteopathic Study Group meeting in the mid-70s, one of the members of the study group asked Rollin Becker a question that had been bothering him since medical school. When looking at histology slides he had wondered how the cells in the middle of the capillary bed got the same nutrition as those around the edges. Dr. Becker used the analogy of a seine lying flat on a beach with each capillary bed represented by a square in the seine, and the capillaries, arterioles, and venules represented by the strings of the seine. The waves bathe the seine as they wash up over it, and again as they flow back. Which one of the cells within any of those squares gets more or less nutrition and disposes of more or less metabolic waste? Because of the seine-like structure, they are all equivalent. The capillaries, arterioles, and venules add nutrients and remove wastes from the interstitial fluid as it passes by. The cells within the capillary beds draw their nutrients from this fluid as it passes by, and dump their wastes into it to be carried off. The waves of interstitial fluid ebb and flow at approximately 10 to 14 times a minute, which is similar to the rate of flow of waves in the ocean.[6] The tide, wave, or cranial rhythmic impulse all refer to the rhythmic motion of the interstitial fluids throughout the body. Sutherland referred to the motion that carried on cellular respiration as the "breath of life."

In other words, the capillary beds are hooked together into one big grid.[7] Closer observation of this same histological section reveals that the individual cells are organized into a matrix, which creates channels by which the nutrient-rich fluids of the body travel to supply all the cells equally, even those farthest from the source. The primary respiratory mechanism pushes fluids into these matrices, creating fluid waves within the body.[8] It is this hydrodynamic fluctuation that nourishes every cell. The cells depend on this tide to avoid the buildup of lactic acids, carbon dioxide, and other metabolic wastes around and in the cells. Twenty percent of the body weight is in the extracellular compartments, which contain approximately 14 liters of fluid that moves between cells and fascial planes.[9]

Rollin Becker, D.O., observed that "Studying the cadaver is like studying a telephone pole to find out how a tree works."[10] This is also true for histology and anatomy as it is taught in schools. You are looking at something dead, pickled, and without motion. What we are dealing with when treating patients, however, is living, so you have to look at the living anatomy. You have to look at the living human body to see what is really happening.

Now visualize an area of dysfunction where the interstitial fluid is not moving. If the matrix is disturbed, the channels cannot function to supply those innermost cells. The individual cell within each capillary bed picks up only the nutrition that can diffuse to it from the capillaries, arterioles, and venules, and disposes of waste in a similar manner. The cells in this area of dysfunction are existing at a lower level of vitality than those in areas of normal function where the interstitial fluid is flowing properly. This area becomes a "dead spot," a place where the hydrodynamic fluctuation is not penetrating. You have an area where there is no motion—somatic dysfunction at the cellular level. Those cells in the center are not getting sufficient nutrients and are not effectively getting rid of their wastes, that is, a site of dysfunction.[11] Hence, the pain in the area of dysfunction results from the buildup of waste products, such as prostaglandins and nitrogenous waste, and hypoxia of the cells. By using manipulation to restore this fluid motion through the area of dysfunction, function can be regained and the stagnating spot revived.

# Fascia

A. T. Still looked to the fascia for the source of disease.[12] Strains in the fascia not only pull bones out of position and impinge on nerves, vessels, and lymphatics; they also impede the flow of the interstitial fluid. At the 1998 Cranial Academy Conference, the osteopathic anatomist Frank Willard, Ph.D., stated that the fascia should be defined and studied as a system unto itself and not simply as an obscuring material hiding more important tissues.[13] Remember that from an embryological standpoint, fascia, bone, and all the connective tissues arise from the mesenchyme.

## *Connective Tissue*

Connective tissue makes up about 16 percent of the body's weight and stores approximately 25 percent of the body's total water. It forms the biological building blocks of the skin, muscles, nerve sheaths, tendons, ligaments, fascia, blood vessels, joint capsules, periosteum, aponeuroses, bones, adipose tissue, and cartilage and the framework for the internal organs.[14] Connective tissue, with a special emphasis on fascia for our purposes here, has unique deformative characteristics.

The fascia derives its unique characteristics from its viscosity and elasticity, both of which are changed by manipulation to reinstate homeostasis in the body. Being viscoelastic in nature, the fascia has both permanent (viscous) and temporary (elastic) deformation characteristics.[15,16] In addition, fascia has a plastic component that allows for permanent elongation and a mechanical component that allows it to contract; thus, the fascia and bones deform in the same four ways. Wolff's law states:

> Every change in form and function of a bone, or in its function alone, is followed by certain definite changes in its internal architecture and secondary alterations in its external conformations, for example, bone is laid down along lines of stress.[17]

This process apparently also applies to the fascia and all connective tissue.

## Crimping

If there are abnormal stresses found in the collagen that makes up the tendons and ligaments, then the tendons and ligaments will be deformed and their basic functions will be affected. Tendons attach muscle fibers to bones and transmit muscle forces, and the ligaments check excess motion of the joints and guide joint motion.[18] Ligaments have a less consistent parallel arrangement of collagen than tendons.[19] The orientation of the ligament takes on an undulating configuration known as the *crimp*, which allows the ligament to work like a spring and which is an essential function of normal ligaments.[20] Upon injury to the ligament, the spring will be straightened, causing the ligament to function improperly.

# Immobilization

Scientific studies have shown that fascia and connective tissue have certain biochemical and physiologic responses to immobilization. Most of the currently available research is on animals, which may limit its application to the human population. Nevertheless, in the studies on animal connective tissues, laboratory animals were immobilized for various periods of time and then examined at different time intervals.[21]

## Biochemical Changes Secondary to Immobilization

1. Fibrofatty infiltrates were found in the capsular folds and recesses, and the longer the joint was immobilized, the greater the amount of infiltration.[22]

2. There was a loss of water and of glycosaminoglycans in the ground substance, a lubricant found between the collagen fibers, which are the primary connective tissue fibers that compose the fascia. Collagen fiber lubrication is associated with the maintenance of a critical interfiber dis-

tance, which has to be maintained between the fibers in order for them to move smoothly. When this distance is not maintained, microadhesions form and new collagen is then laid down in a haphazard manner.[23]

3.  Immobilization for greater than 12 weeks resulted in an overall loss of collagen since its rate of degradation exceeded its rate of synthesis under these circumstances.[24]

4.  Joint contracture occurred as the result of remodeling and shortening of connective tissues when connective tissue is immobilized in the presence of inflammatory exudates. When a limb is immobilized in the absence of inflammatory exudates, no contracture occurs. In addition, biochemical changes were noted.[25,26]

### *Physiological Changes Secondary to Immobilization*

1.  The force needed to move an immobilized joint was ten times that of a normal joint. After several repetitions, the amount of force required to move the immobilized joint was reduced to three times that of a normal joint. Over time, the joint will usually regain normal joint mobility.[27]

2.  Manipulation of experimentally immobilized rat knees by either high velocity techniques or range of motion resulted in the rupture of macroadhesions and the restoration of partial joint mobility. Movement restores the normal histological makeup of the connective tissue, but the chances of obtaining optimum results decreases as the immobilization period increases.[28]

3.  All periarticular connective tissues responded in the same manner. Ligament and capsule surrounding the fascia all have the same basic response to immobilization. Manual manipulation of the tissues causes a reversal of effects, provided manipulation was done within three months of immobilization.[17,25]

# Plastic Bags

Every cell in the body is surrounded by fascia that fuse together to make bigger sheets of fascia. Eventually, these fuse together to form tendons and ligaments. When you look at the smallest fibers of a muscle, it is still surrounded by fascia. It is like plastic bags within plastic bags within plastic bags. It is through pressure on these "plastic bags" that we are causing a change in the body.

Pascal's law states that "Pressure applied to a liquid at rest from any point is transmitted equally in all directions."[29] The human body consists of many closed fluid systems like the plastic bags that respond exactly as predicted by Pascal's principle, that is, an increase in the pressure of fluid in one of the plastic bags will distribute its pressure to other portions of the body.

When teaching ligamentous articular strain, we often have one person place a hand on the anterior cervical fascia (Sibson's fascia) on the right while another person places a hand on the left pelvic diaphragm. One presses while the other feels the pressure at the other end, and vice versa. The connection is very direct. This simple exercise illustrates the essence of Pascal's principle as applied to the human body and shows how ligamentous articular strain is initiated through external force.

We believe that manipulation of the body can even affect us on the cellular level. The effects of the hydrodynamic fluctuation of body fluids restore motion and life to "dead spots," or somatic dysfunctions, changing the structure of the tissues. Research has shown that changes in the structure of the tissues of the body alters the structure of the endoskeleton of the cell,[30] which in turn can actually alter gene expression and cellular metabolism. Therefore, we believe that we can bring about significant change on all levels by manipulating the tissues of the body.

We know that there is some cerebrospinal fluid uptake by the lymphatics. As Dr. Still stated, "Cerebrospinal fluid is one of the highest known elements that is contained in the human body and unless the brain furnishes this fluid in abundance, a disabled condition of the body will remain."[31]

Therefore, the cerebrospinal fluid can be used as a "penetrating oil," as Dr. Sutherland called it, and make changes on the cellular level using the cranial rhythmic impulse (CRI).

> I want to call your attention to the benefits of managing the fluctuation of the cerebrospinal fluid when treating chronic lesion in the spinal column. I call it "penetrating oil" for use on old rusty lesions. … When it has had time to work, he takes only his fingers to turn the nut and the bolt and does not injure either the threads of the nut or the bolt. By bringing the Tide down to that short rhythmic period and to that important interchange between all the fluids of the body, you can lubricate those chronic situations gradually so that they return to normal functional conditions. Fibrosis also fades out, and normal muscle tissue reappears in due time.[32]

In *Osteopathy in the Cranial Field*, Harold Magoun described the circulation and the hydrodynamic action of the cerebrospinal fluid,[33] which is due in part to the inherent motility of the central nervous system. The cerebral spinal fluid is produced on the floor of the third ventricle of the brain and flows out through the nervous system. It then exits "by way of Pacchionian bodies in the venous sinuses, out along the cranial and spinal perineural spaces, and also through the hollow collagen fibers of the fascia into the lymphatic system"[34] to mix with the other interstitial fluids of the body; thus, the entire body is moving with the "breath of life." The floor of the third ventricle is thus like a spring coming up in the floor of an ocean that is ebbing and flowing. As Royder explained:

> The circulation of cerebrospinal fluid flows from its point of origin, in the choroid plexuses in the ventricles, around and through the brain and down the spinal cord. The cerebrospinal fluid not only moves down the spinal cord but also down the axons, contributing to the transneural axoplasmic flow.[35]

This concept is echoed in the osteopathic literature:

> Every organ in the body exhibits the phenomenon of pulsations or rhythmic action which is incessantly active, dynamic, highly mobile; resulting in forward, backwards, sideways, and rotational fluid movement.[28]

These palpable pulsations induced by the primary respiratory mechanism can thus produce extracellular fluid movement throughout the body.

These pulsations appear to be ubiquitous. They propel the extracellular fluids into and across the semipermeable membranes of cells everywhere and deliver nutrients and remove metabolic waste products even from synovial spaces, bursae, and other nonvascular compartments. Every cell membrane of the body is continuously and rhythmically bathed with these essential fluids in a fashion similar to the ebb and flow of the ocean upon the beach.

# Vector of Injury

Another factor we must consider is the vector of injury. First, we must define our terms. In mathematics, a vector denotes a directed line segment with a certain magnitude and direction. A vector of injury is the firm or hard tract left through the body after a vector of force has passed through it. These areas are palpable and are the areas of dysfunction. For example, a football player is struck in the side of the chest with an opponent's helmet. By having the patient lie on his side and compressing at the point of injury toward the table with the palm of the hand, the practitioner can locate the exact direction and magnitude of the vector of injury. It will feel like a section of broomstick between the palm and the treatment table oriented along the direction of impact *(Figure 3.1)*.

Vectors of injury can be treated by either indirect or direct methods. Whenever possible, indirect methods are preferable because they are usually less painful. A ligamentous articular release technique using an indirect method would be indicated for treating the above mentioned football injury. This would be accomplished by compressing the ribs medially (disengagement) in as far as they were compressed by the original blow (exaggeration) and maintaining that pressure until a release occurs (balance). The ribs

**Figure 3.1** Vector

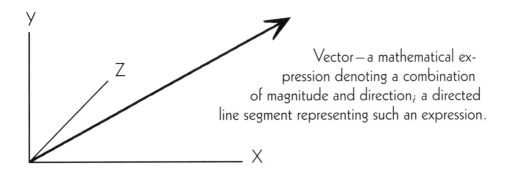

Vector—a mathematical expression denoting a combination of magnitude and direction; a directed line segment representing such an expression.

will move in slightly farther, and then expand outward as you slowly release the pressure.

Using the direct method technique would involve grabbing the injured ribs, if possible, and pulling them back out. However, for this particular injury, that would be virtually impossible. A more practical example of the direct method is as follows. Suppose that the first rib is elevated, resulting in spasms in the scalene muscles that pull the first rib superiorly out of its socket at the costovertebral junction. A technique for treating this using a direct method is to contact the first rib at its head and apply pressure inferiorly (disengagement), maintaining firm balanced pressure inferiorly on top of the head of the first rib until it releases and slips inferiorly back into socket. Note that in this technique there is no exaggeration of the dysfunction, which is true of most of the techniques using the direct method.

In general, indirect techniques are like pushing on the tail of the vector of injury. By contrast, direct techniques are like pulling on the tail of the vector of injury or pushing on the point of the arrow.

# Conclusion

Fluid dynamics, joint physiology, fascia, and vectors of injury may look on the surface to be unrelated, but, on a deeper level, are found to be closely connected. As osteopaths we are interested in continuously advancing our skills and studying the interrelatedness of biomechanics. As you expand your knowledge of osteopathy, you will move from a view of the human body as a skeleton, with other tissues hanging on as it were, to a view of the body as a moving, living organism with a skeleton found within it. As a result, your attention will move from bones and joints to the fascia and fluid dynamics. It is important to understand the scientific principles upon which these techniques are based in order to apply them most successfully. If you understand the principles, you can then create your own techniques.

Look at a somatic dysfunction as an impediment to the flow of the interstitial fluid. The fluid moves around the vectors of injury and other areas of dysfunction like a stream flows around a stone. The goal of your treatment is to remove the stone and let the stream flow through unimpeded. Take that which you palpate as hard and make it soft. When you feel the flow come through the dysfunctional area, your treatment of that area is complete.

1   Sutherland WG. *Teachings in the Science of Osteopathy*, ed. Anne Wales, D.O. Rudra Press, 1990: 234.

2   Frank C, Amiel D, Akeson W. Normal ligaments properties and ligament healing. *Clinical Orthopedics & Related Research* 1985; 196:15–25.

3   Lippincott HA. "The Osteopathic Technique of Wm. G. Sutherland, D.O." in *1949 Yearbook of the Academy of Applied Osteopathy.* Reprint, Indianapolis, IN: American Academy of Osteopathy.

4   Ibid., 2.

5   Sutherland, *Teachings in the Science of Osteopathy,* 186.

6   Magoun HI. *Osteopathy in the Cranial Field,* 3rd ed. Indianapolis, IN: The Cranial Academy, 1976: 25.

7   Ward RC., ed. *Foundations for Osteopathic Medicine.* Baltimore, MD: Williams and Wilkins, 1997: 31.

8   Magoun, *Osteopathy in the Cranial Field,* 23, defines the Primary Respiratory Mechanism as a unit of physiological function which includes the following five phenomena: 1) inherent motility of the brain and spinal cord; 2) fluctuation of the cerebrospinal fluid; 3) mobility of the intracranial and intraspinal membranes; 4) articular mobility of the cranial bones; and 5) involuntary mobility of the sacrum between the ilia.

9   Frank, "Normal ligaments properties," 15–25.

10   Roland Becker, speaking at a Dallas Osteopathic Study Group Meeting, date uncertain.

11   Van Buskirk RL. Nociceptive reflexes and the somatic dysfunction: a model. *Journal of the American Osteopathic Association* 1990; 90(9): 792–805.

12   Still AT. *Philosophy of Osteopathy.* Kirksville, MO: The Journal Printing Company, 1899: 4.

13   Transcripton of notes taken at Cranial Academy Conference, 1998.

14   Ham AW. *Histology.* Philadelphia, PA: JB Lippincott, 1979: 210–19.

15   Stromberg DD, Weiderhielm DA. Viscoelastic description of a collagenous tissue in simple elongation. *Journal of Applied Physiology* 1969; 26:857–862.

16   Hooley CJ, McCrum NG, Cohen RE. The visceoelastic deformation of tendon. *Journal of Biomechanics* 1980; 13:521–528.

17   *American Osteopathic Association Yearbook and Directory of Osteopathic Physicians.* Chicago, IL: American Osteopathic Association, 1998: 773.

18  Frankel VH, Nordin M. *Basic Biomechanics of the Skeletal System.* Philadelphia, PA: Lea and Febiger, 1980: 56:87–110.

19  Kennedy JC, Hawkins RJ, Willis RB, Danylchuck KD. Tension studies of human knee ligaments, yield point, ultimate failure and disruption of the cruciate and tibial collateral ligaments. *Journal of Bone and Joint Surgery* 1976; 58:A350–55.

20  Frank, "Normal ligaments properties," 15–25.

21  Woo S, Matthew JV, Akeson WH, Amiel D, Convery FR. Connective tissue response to immobility. *Arthritis & Rheumatism* 1975; 18:257–64.

22  Akeson WH, Woo S, Amiel D, Coutts RD, Daniel D. The connective tissue response to immobilization: biochemical changes in periarticular connective tissue of the rabbit knee. *Clinical Orthopedics & Related Research* 1973; 93:356–62.

23  Akeson WH, Amiel D, LaViolette D, Secrist D. The connective tissue response to immobility: an accelerated aging response. *Experimental Gerontology* 1968; 3(4):289–301.

24  Akeson WH, Amiel D. Immobility effects of synovial joints: the pathomechanics of joint contracture. *Biorheology* 1980; 17:95–110.

25  Akeson WH, Arniel D, LaViolette D. The connective tissue response to immobility: a study of the chondroitin-4 and 6-sulfate dermatan sulfate changes in periarticular connective tissue of control and immobilized knees of dogs. *Clinical Orthopaedics & Related Research* 1967; 51:183–97.

26  Amiel D, Akeson WH, Harwood FL, Frank CB. Stress deprivation effect on metabolic turnover of medial collateral ligament collagen. *Clinical Orthopedics & Related Research* 1983; 172:265–70.

27  Evans E, Egger G, Butler JA, Blumb, J. Experimental immobilization and mobilization of rat knee joints. *The Journal of Bone and Joint Surgery* (American Edition) 1960; 42A(5):737–58.

28  Ibid.

29  *Stedman's Medical Dictionary,* 26th ed. Baltimore, MD: Williams & Wilkins, 1995: 942.

30  Chen CS, Ingber DE. Tensegrity and mechanoregulation: from skeleton to cytoskeleton. *Osteoarthritis Cartilage* 1999; 7(1):81–94.

31  Still AT, *The Philosophy and Mechanical Principles of Osteopathy.* Kansas City, MO: Hudson Kimberly Publishing Company, 1902: 44.

32  Sutherland, *Teachings in Science of Osteopathy,* 185-86.

33  Magoun, *Osteopathy in the Cranial Field,* 24.

34  Ibid., 20.

35  Royder J, Fluid hydraulics in human physiology. *American Academy of Osteopathy Journal* 1997; 7(2):11-17.

# General Osteopathic Techniques

# CHAPTER FOUR

# The Lower Extremities

The lower extremities are among the most important structures of the body and yet are often overlooked. Each lower extremity contains two of the major transverse planes in the body, that is, the foot and the knee. If these transverse planes are dysfunctional, they can act as baffles,[1] which may result in a blockage of fluid flow from the lower extremity, producing both local and systemic effects. Another neglected aspect of the lower extremities is the connection between their fascial compartments and muscles and the lower back. For example, it is not rare for lower back pain to be due to a dysfunction of the popliteal fascia.

In addition, as the lower extremities are the foundation for the rest of the body, an imbalance in either of the lower extremities can affect the musculature of the trunk or the viscera. The effects of lower extremity problems can be far reaching. For example, arrhythmia can occur after a knee injury due to the center of gravity moving forward, causing the pelvis to tilt and resulting in mild scoliosis. This in turn can lead to an impingement of cranial nerve XI (vagus), which innervates the heart. Treatment of all the dysfunctional structures, starting with the knee, can resolve the arrhythmia.

---

[1] William Garner Sutherland called the LAS techniques he used general osteopathic techniques.

[2] This concept appears again in Chapter 11. Briefly, baffles are obstructions to flow within a structure. In a gas tank baffles keep the fluid from sloshing around. However, for optimal health fluids should slosh around the body. Therefore if structures are acting as baffles, we try and help them turn back into diaphragms. You want everything working together and everything moving.

# Foot

## *Plantar Fascia*

TECHNIQUE: Supine direct myofascial release

SYMPTOMS/DIAGNOSIS: Pain on the bottom of the foot, heel spurs, or plantar fasciitis

PATIENT: Supine

PHYSICIAN: Seated at the foot of the table

PROCEDURE: Your thumbs are crossed and the pads are pressed into the plantar fascia at the level of the tarsal-metatarsal junctions with your fingers interlaced across the dorsum of the foot. The pads of the thumbs press in the direction the thumbs are pointed, that is, toward either side of the foot and slightly toward the toes, and are taken to a point of balanced tension. Once a release occurs, your thumb tips seem to slip across the fascia. Repeat the same procedure with the toes in plantar flexion. Once that release occurs, repeat the procedure with the toes in dorsiflexion. The treatment of the plantar fascia is complete once you have accomplished all three releases.

**Figure 4.1** Plantar fascia technique

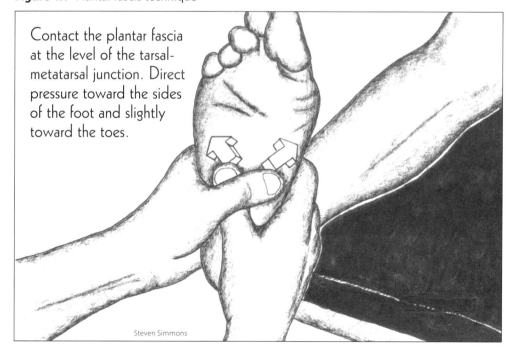

Contact the plantar fascia at the level of the tarsal-metatarsal junction. Direct pressure toward the sides of the foot and slightly toward the toes.

Steven Simmons

**Figure 4.2**  Plantar flexion

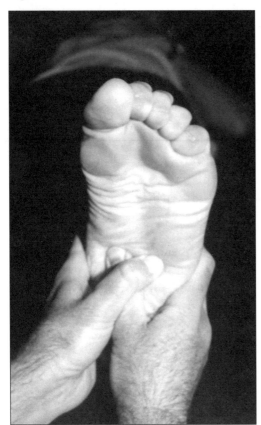

Instruct the patient to "step on the gas," forcing the foot into plantar flexion.

**Figure 4.3**  Dorsiflexion

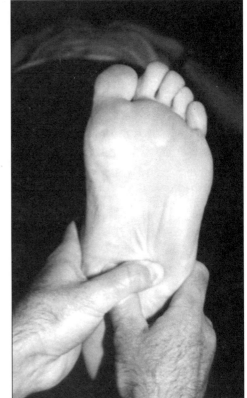

Instruct the patient to bend the toes toward the head.

## *Metatarsals, Tarsals, and Toes*

TECHNIQUE: Supine indirect ligamentous articular release

SYMPTOMS/DIAGNOSIS: Pain in the middle of the foot or in the toes

PATIENT: Supine with the heels on the table

PHYSICIAN: Standing at the foot of the table, facing toward the head of the table

PROCEDURE: While bending forward above the patient's foot, wrap both your hands around the affected foot from either side with the distal toes imbedded in the palms of your hands and the foot drawn into slight plantar flexion by contracting your fingers under the distal metatarsals. The thumbs are on the dorsum of the foot. With your weight, compress the phalanges, metatarsals, and tarsals directly into the table, balancing on top of the rod-like vector force felt between your hands and the table. When the release occurs, the tissue softens under your fingers.

**Figure 4.4** Metatarsals, tarsals, and toes technique

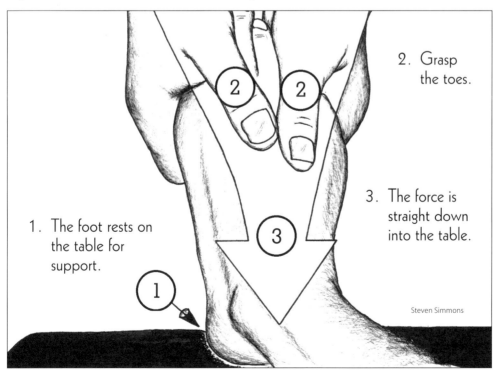

2. Grasp the toes.

3. The force is straight down into the table.

1. The foot rests on the table for support.

Steven Simmons

**Figure 4.5** Metatarsals hand placement (plantar view)

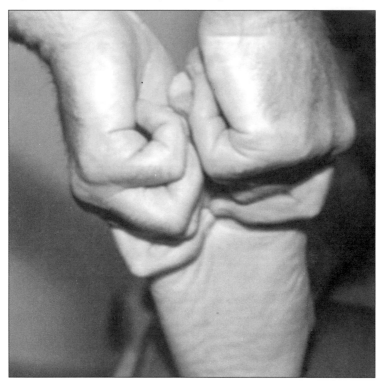

## *Calcaneus (Bootjack Technique)*

TECHNIQUE: Supine combination ligamentous articular release (direct on calcaneus and indirect on forefoot)

SYMPTOMS/DIAGNOSIS: Heel or foot pain, or heel spurs

PATIENT: Supine

PHYSICIAN: Standing on the same side of the table as the affected heel, facing toward the foot of the table

PROCEDURE: Externally rotate and abduct the patient's femur and flex the knee. Place the posterior distal humerus of the arm you have closest to the table across the patient's distal femur just above the popliteal fossa. Your humerus and the patient's femur should be approximately 90° to each other. Grasp their calcaneus with your thumb and the proximal interphalangeal joint of the bent index finger of the same hand. Lean toward the patient's head, carrying the knee into deeper flexion to exert traction on the heel. While carrying the heel distally, balance the front of the foot with your other hand. Grasp under the distal first metatarsal with the thumb of that hand, the fingertips wrapping around the little toe and lateral aspect of the foot.

Balance the tension in the metatarsals and tarsals between your two hands while you carry the calcaneus inferiorly, away from the head. When the release at the heel occurs, it feels like your thumb and index finger slip off the calcaneus. You will also feel a softening in the forefoot when it releases. Both releases may occur at the same time or independently.

**Figure 4.6** Bootjack technique

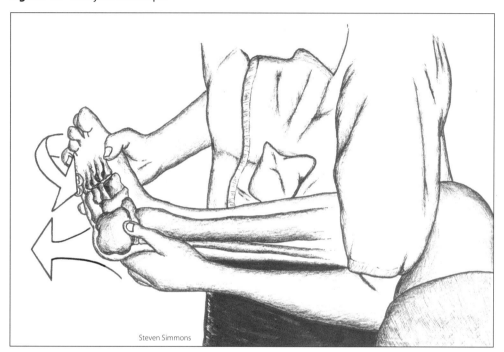

Steven Simmons

# Ankle

## *Unstable Ankle*

The function of the ankle is closely tied to the function of the knee. When the fibular head is subluxed at the knee, the head rides on the rim of its socket. This drives the distal end inferiorly and makes the ankle joint not level, that is, the fibular side is more inferior. As a result, the ankle mortise is unstable, and the patient chronically rolls off the outside of the foot, respraining the ankle. To stabilize an ankle, the fibula must be returned to its socket at the knee. Utilize the fibular head technique, which is described later in this chapter, to treat the unstable ankle. Once the fibula is returned to its normal position and the ankle mortise is level, the ligaments can begin their three month healing process. If it is not reinjured, the ankle will once again be stable.

## *Talus Anterior*

TECHNIQUE: Supine indirect ligamentous articular release

SYMPTOMS/DIAGNOSIS: Ankle pain or difficulty dorsiflexing the foot, such as when going up or down stairs. This can be diagnosed by sweeping your palpating thumb down the front of the tibia. The anterior talus feels like a shelf in front of the tibia.

PATIENT: Supine with the heel on the table

PHYSICIAN: Standing at the side of the table, at the level of the affected ankle

PROCEDURE: Place the palm of your distal hand across the distal tibia with the hypothenar side of the palm located within one-fourth to one-half inch of the talus. Compress the tibia directly down toward the table. You should feel tension coming up through the heel and directly through the tibiotalar joint. Roll the lower leg slightly internally or externally to bring the force to its exact balance point (where the tension is most intense). It will feel like you have met a barrier with the rotation. Your other hand can be placed over the top of the treating hand to reinforce it. The amount of pressure will be in the 10 to 40 pound range. Maintain this balance point until the release occurs, at which time the palpable tension will soften and the lower leg will roll through the barrier. Slowly remove the pressure, allowing the tibia to move back over the talus in an anterior direction. The treatment is complete. Remember to recheck the foot to see that the shelf- or step-like projection is gone.

**Figure 4.5** Metatarsals hand placement (plantar view)

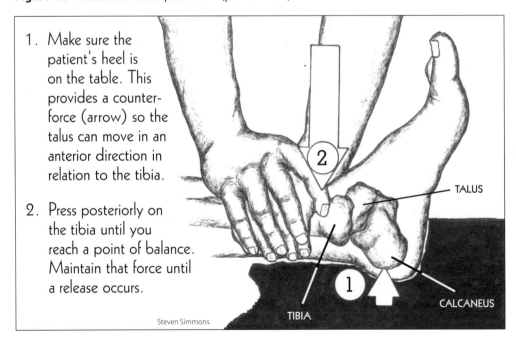

1. Make sure the patient's heel is on the table. This provides a counter-force (arrow) so the talus can move in an anterior direction in relation to the tibia.

2. Press posteriorly on the tibia until you reach a point of balance. Maintain that force until a release occurs.

Steven Simmons

TALUS

CALCANEUS

TIBIA

# *Talus Posterior*

TECHNIQUE: Supine indirect ligamentous articular release

SYMPTOMS/DIAGNOSIS: Ankle pain or difficulty plantar flexing the foot (such as when going up or down stairs). The cause is posterior subluxation of the talus on the tibia. This can be diagnosed by drawing the thumb superiorly on the anterior tibiotalar junction and feeling a small shelf-like projection of the distal tibia that has shifted anteriorly on the talus.

PATIENT: Supine with the heel just off end of table. The heel should clear the end of the table by approximately one inch.

PHYSICIAN: Standing at the foot of the table, facing the head of the table

PROCEDURE: Using the table to support the distal tibia, carry the foot toward the floor. To accomplish this, bend forward above the patient's foot, wrapping both your hands around the foot from the sides with the distal toes imbedded in the palms of your hands and the foot drawn into slight flexion by contracting your fingers under the distal metatarsals. Your thumbs are on the dorsum of the foot. Apply pressure downward to the entire foot, directly past the end of the table toward the floor to a balance point. When the release occurs, it feels like the foot shifts more posteriorly on the ankle. Slowly decrease the downward pressure, allowing the foot to move anteriorly on the ankle joint and to recenter itself.

**Figure 4.8** Talus posterior technique

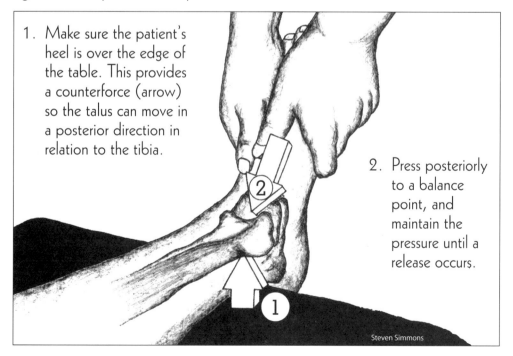

1. Make sure the patient's heel is over the edge of the table. This provides a counterforce (arrow) so the talus can move in a posterior direction in relation to the tibia.

2. Press posteriorly to a balance point, and maintain the pressure until a release occurs.

Steven Simmons

# The Leg

## *Dorsiflexors of the Foot and Pretibial Fascia*

TECHNIQUE: Supine direct myofascial release

SYMPTOMS/DIAGNOSIS: Pain down the front of the lower leg, shin splints, or dorsi-cramping of toes. The most common type of shin splints can be attributed to strains of the pretibial fascia and spasm of the dorsiflexors of the foot.

PATIENT: Supine

PHYSICIAN: Standing, facing the side of the table, at the level of the lower leg

PROCEDURE: Place the pad of the thumb of your more distal hand on the anterior surface of the dorsiflexor muscles and pretibial fascia just lateral to the tibia. Find the tightest point in the fascia and muscle, and maintain a balanced compressive force (in the range of 20 to 40 pounds of pressure) medially and posteriorly with your thumb, parallel and just lateral to the tibia, until you feel a release. Reinforce your distal thumb with your more proximal thumb to avoid fatigue of the treating thumb. When the release occurs, the hard spasm will melt—the muscle and fascia have relaxed. This treats the dorsiflexor muscles of the foot and toes.

**Figure 4.9**  Dorsiflexors of the foot and pretibial fascia technique

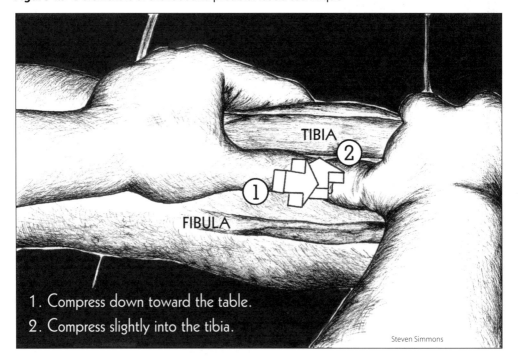

TIBIA

②

①

FIBULA

1. Compress down toward the table.
2. Compress slightly into the tibia.

Steven Simmons

## *Plantar Flexors of the Foot and Calf*

TECHNIQUE: Supine direct myofascial release

SYMPTOMS/DIAGNOSIS: Calf pain, cramping of the foot, and/or cramping of the plantar aspect of the toes

PATIENT: Supine

PHYSICIAN: Sitting at the side of the table just distal to patient's calf, facing the head of the table

PROCEDURE: With the fingers bent, line up the fingertips of both your hands side by side with your eight fingers under and transverse to the gastrocnemius and soleus muscles, allowing the weight of the leg to rest on your fingertips. Press into the tight flexor muscle, which feels like a tight guitar string, with the finger that is directly under the tight spot. With the weight of the leg applying the needed pressure, slightly draw that finger inferiorly toward the foot. Maintain that balanced tension until the release occurs.

**Figure 4.10**  Plantar flexors of the foot and calf technique

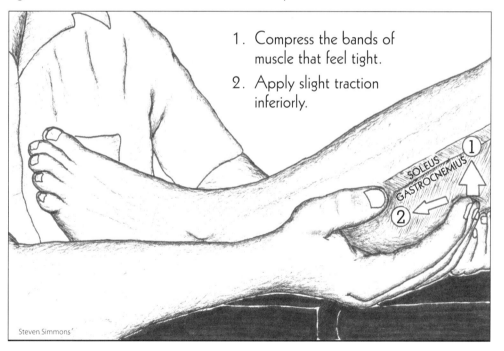

# Knee

## *Fibular Head*

TECHNIQUE: Supine direct ligamentous articular release

SYMPTOMS/DIAGNOSIS: Posterior and lateral knee pain or unstable ankle with chronic spraining of the ankle. The latter is a result of an unstable ankle mortise with the fibula displaced at the knee.

PATIENT: Supine

PHYSICIAN: Seated, facing the side of the table at the level of the affected knee

PROCEDURE: Flex the hip and the knee to approximately 90°. Slightly externally rotate the femur. With the arm closest to the patient's head, bend your elbow to 90° and prop it on the table, making a vertical pedestal with your forearm and thumb. With the pad of this thumb, push the posterior superior portion of the fibular head inferiorly toward the foot. The distal hand inverts the foot and slightly rotates the foot medially. This pulls on the distal end of the fibula. Balance the connective tissue surrounding both ends of the fibula and the interosseous membrane between the tibia and fibula until a release occurs. The fibular head moves inferiorly and anteriorly and slides back into its socket.

**Figure 4.11**  Fibula technique hand placements

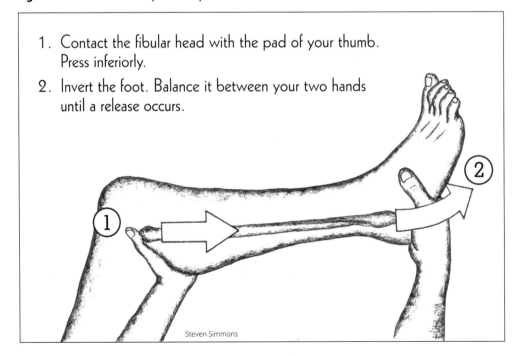

1. Contact the fibular head with the pad of your thumb. Press inferiorly.

2. Invert the foot. Balance it between your two hands until a release occurs.

Steven Simmons

## *Lateral (Fibular) Collateral Ligament of the Knee*

TECHNIQUE: Supine combination ligamentous articular release (direct on the lateral collateral ligament and indirect on the medial collateral ligament)

SYMPTOMS/DIAGNOSIS: Pain on the lateral aspect of the knee from a strained lateral collateral ligament

PATIENT: Supine

PHYSICIAN: Seated, facing the side of the table at the level of the knee

PROCEDURE: Externally rotate and abduct the hip on the affected side. Bring the knee into approximately 90° of flexion. (The patient's other leg remains straight.) With the hand closest to the end of the table, grasp the patient's foot with your fingers in the instep and your thumb on the lateral dorsum of the foot. The hypothenar eminence supports the lateral aspect of the calcaneus, and the thenar eminence is directly inferior to the distal fibula. Prop that elbow on the table, and without supporting the knee with the other hand, allow the knee to drop laterally toward the floor. With your hand holding the foot, invert the foot at the ankle and internally rotate it (which slightly internally rotates the lower leg). Draw the foot inferiorly, straightening the knee while maintaining the balanced tension across the lateral collateral ligament. The hand on the foot monitors the tension on the knee. When the knee catches at a barrier, maintain balanced tension at that barrier or still point until a release occurs and the knee straightens further.

**Figure 4.13** Lateral collateral ligament set-up

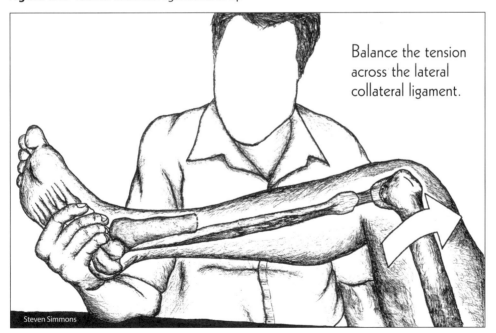

Balance the tension across the lateral collateral ligament.

Steven Simmons

There may be multiple barriers. Maintain steady tension against each barrier encountered until the knee straightens completely. Once the knee has completely straightened, the lateral collateral ligament has returned to its normal physiologic condition and the femur internally rotates to align with the tibia.

**Figure 4.14** Lateral collateral ligament technique

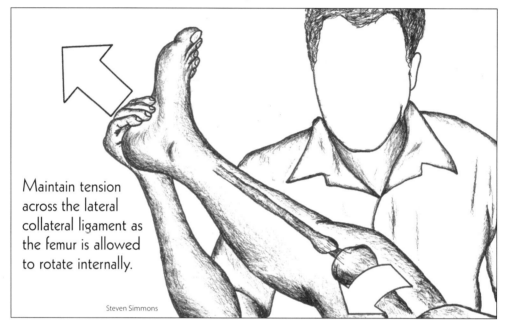

Maintain tension across the lateral collateral ligament as the femur is allowed to rotate internally.

Steven Simmons

## *Medial Collateral Ligament*

TECHNIQUE: Supine combination ligamentous articular release (direct on the medial collateral ligament and indirect on the lateral collateral ligament)

SYMPTOMS/DIAGNOSIS: Pain on the medial aspect of the knee as a result of a strained medial collateral ligament

PATIENT: Supine

PHYSICIAN: Sitting just beyond the corner of the foot of the table on the same side as the affected knee, facing the head of the table

PROCEDURE: Grasp the foot with both hands. Your lateral hand grasps the calcaneus with the fingers on the medial aspect and the thenar eminence on the lateral aspect. Your medial hand grasps the forefoot with the distal end of the first metatarsal in that palm. The hip is flexed and adducted, causing the femur to internally rotate. The knee is bent approximately 90° and is now above the opposite femur. With both hands on the foot, externally rotate the foot and attempt to straighten the leg. Draw the foot inferiorly, straightening the knee while maintaining the balanced tension across the medial collateral ligament. When the knee catches at a barrier, maintain balanced tension at that barrier or still point until the knee straightens further. There may be multiple barriers. Maintain steady pressure against each barrier encountered until the knee straightens completely. When this has occurred, the medial collateral ligament has returned to its normal physiologic condition and the femur externally rotates to align with the tibia.

**Figure 4.15** Medial collateral ligament set-up

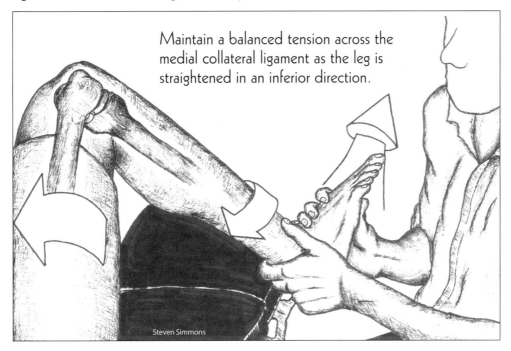

**Figure 4.16** Medial collateral ligament technique

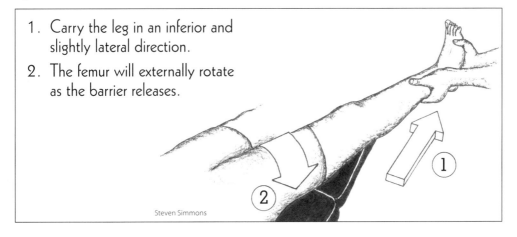

## *Popliteal Fascia*

TECHNIQUE: Supine direct myofascial release

SYMPTOMS/DIAGNOSIS: Pain behind the knee or Baker's cyst

PATIENT: Supine

PHYSICIAN: Seated at the side of the table inferior to the patient's knee, facing the head of the table

PROCEDURE: With the patient's leg relaxed, place your fingertips just above the popliteal fossa. The fingers of both hands are bent with the lateral fingernails of your little fingers and ring fingers touching and the heels of your hands approximately three inches apart. The fingers will form a plough- or wedge-like shape. Grasp the tissue under your fingertips and draw them inferiorly toward the foot. If resistance is met, maintain balanced tension inferiorly and anteriorly until this barrier "melts" and your fingers slide inferiorly with the popliteal fascia melting ahead of the little fingers.

**Figure 4.17** Popliteal fascia technique

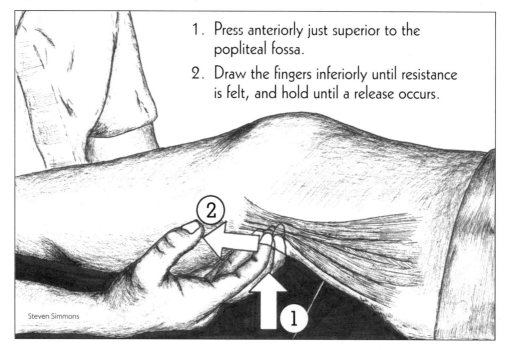

1. Press anteriorly just superior to the popliteal fossa.
2. Draw the fingers inferiorly until resistance is felt, and hold until a release occurs.

Steven Simmons

## *Meniscus*

TECHNIQUE: Supine direct ligamentous articular release

SYMPTOMS/DIAGNOSIS: Pain in the knee, quite often anterior and inferior to the patella, and either lateral or medial. There may be pain deep in the middle of the knee.

PATIENT: Supine with legs straight and relaxed

PHYSICIAN: Sitting at the side of the table inferior to patient's knee, facing the head of the table

PROCEDURE: Once all the strains in the popliteal fascia have been released, palpate the back of the knee for any firm or tender lumps (posteriorly subluxed menisci). A lump that is found toward the medial popliteal fossa is a posteriorly subluxed medial meniscus, while a lump that is found toward the lateral popliteal fossa is a posteriorly subluxed lateral meniscus. If either condition or a combination of both conditions is encountered, use the tip of the pad of the middle finger of your dominant hand reinforced with the pad of the middle finger of your other hand to maintain steady balanced pressure anteriorly on the meniscus until it slips back into its normal position and the lump disappears.

**Figure 4.18**  Meniscus technique

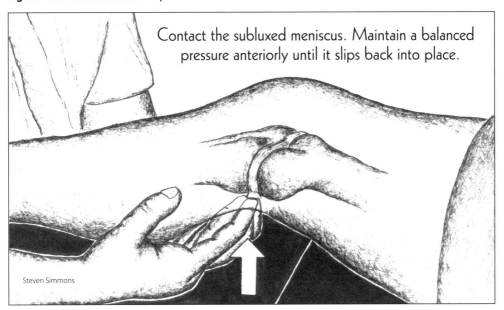

Contact the subluxed meniscus. Maintain a balanced pressure anteriorly until it slips back into place.

Steven Simmons

## *Cruciate Ligaments*

TECHNIQUE: Supine indirect ligamentous articular release

SYMPTOMS/DIAGNOSIS: Pain or swelling in the knee or knee hyperextension. The pain in the knee often occurs when climbing or descending stairs or standing up from a seated position. These symptoms may be a result of a strained anterior or posterior cruciate ligament. The tibial tuberosity is not centered below the midline of the patella, that is, the tibia is either externally or internally rotated on the femur.

PATIENT: Supine

PHYSICIAN: Standing at the side of the table, facing the patient's knee

PROCEDURE: With the hand closest to the patient's head, grasp the thigh approximately five inches above the knee to stabilize the femur. With your other hand, grasp the lower leg approximately four inches below the knee. Press down on the tibia and femur, then compress your hands toward each other. With the femur stabilized, first rotate the tibia laterally, then medially, to evaluate in which direction it most easily moves. Maintain the rotation in that direction. Maintain a balance point on all three forces—pressure down, compression together, and rotation of the tibia—until the release occurs and the lower leg rotates slightly further in the direction in which the rotation was maintained. When you slowly decrease the rotation and compression, the knee will return to its normal physiologic position, and the tide, that is, the cranial rhythmic impulse (discussed in Chapter 3), will flow through the knee. Reevaluate the centering of the tibial tubercle, which will have moved toward the midline of the patella. Note that the transverse ligament of the knee will correct itself when you have treated the strained cruciate ligaments.

**Figure 4.19** Cruciate ligaments technique

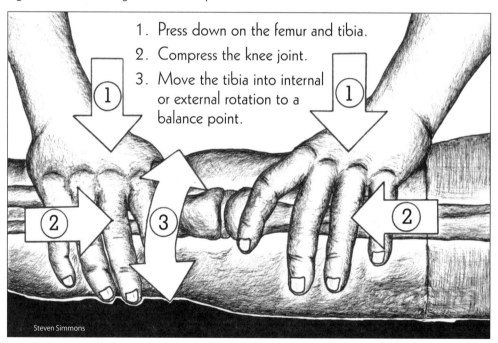

# The Thigh Region

## *Tensor Fascia Latae*

TECHNIQUE: Supine direct myofascial release

SYMPTOMS/DIAGNOSIS: Pain in the lateral groin area on flexing the thigh. Pain is just superior and anterior to the greater trochanter of the femur.

PATIENT: Supine

PHYSICIAN: Standing, facing the affected hip

PROCEDURE: Locate the center of the spasm in the tensor fascia latae just anterior and superior to the greater trochanter. Contact the strain with your thumb and push posteriorly and medially, maintaining steady balanced pressure, until a release occurs.

**Figure 4.20**  Fascia latae technique

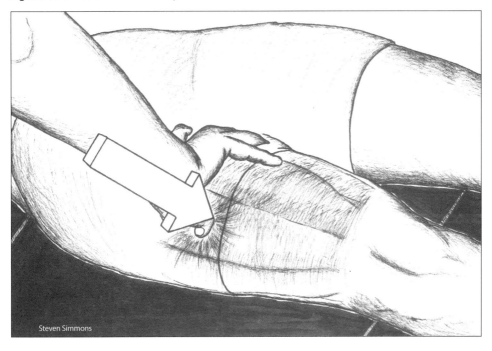

Steven Simmons

## *Iliotibial Tract (Band)*

TECHNIQUE: Supine direct myofascial release

SYMPTOMS/DIAGNOSIS: Pain down the lateral aspect of the thigh

PATIENT: Supine

PHYSICIAN: Standing or seated, facing the affected thigh

PROCEDURE: Locate the tightest point in the tract along the lateral aspect of the thigh. Using the pad of your dominant thumb, reinforced by your other thumb, press medially and posteriorly on this point. Maintain this balanced pressure until a release occurs. The pressure is in the 10- to 30-pound range.

**Figure 4.21**  Iliotibial tract technique

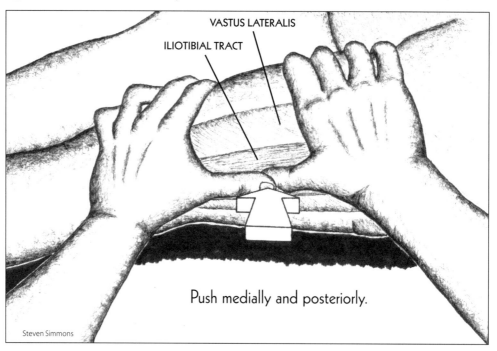

Push medially and posteriorly.

Steven Simmons

# Adductors of the Femur

## *Pectineus, Adductor Brevis, Adductor Longus, Adductor Magnus, and Gracilis*

TECHNIQUE: Supine direct myofascial release

SYMPTOMS/DIAGNOSIS: Groin pain or pain in the medial thigh as a result of strained groin muscles. The foot on the affected side will be relatively internally rotated (pigeon-toed).

PATIENT: Supine with the leg slightly abducted

PHYSICIAN: Standing on the opposite side of the table from the medial aspect of the affected thigh

PROCEDURE: Locate the specific muscle or muscles that are in spasm on the upper medial aspect of the thigh. With the pad of your thumb on the tightest point of spasm, press toward the femur superiorly, slightly posteriorly, and laterally. Maintain this steady, balanced, perpendicular pressure to the fibers until the muscle relaxes. This area is very tender, and if you let the patient know that you are aware of this tenderness, he or she can better tolerate the discomfort until a release occurs. Treat each muscle that is in spasm. When the groin muscles and external hip rotators are all balanced and the patient is fully relaxed, both feet will turn out equally.

**Figure 4.22** Adductors of the femur technique

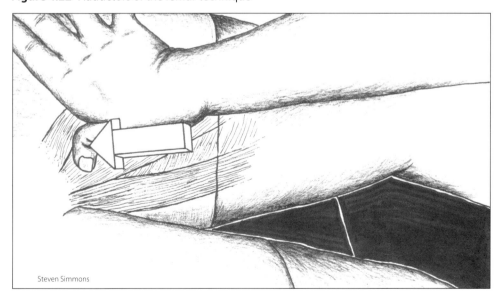

Steven Simmons

# External Hip Rotators and Abductors of the Femur

## *Gluteus Minimus, Superior Gemellus, Obturator Internus, Inferior Gemellus, Quadratus Femoris, Piriformis, and Gluteus Medius*

SYMPTOMS/DIAGNOSIS: Sciatica, hip pain, pain in the gluteal area, or pain down the back of the leg

PATIENT: Lateral recumbent position with the affected hip up and both hips flexed to approximately 90 to 120°. Knees bent to approximately 90°. The patient's back is approximately four inches from the edge of the table.

PHYSICIAN: Standing behind patient at the level of patient's hip, facing the table

## *Gluteus Minimus*

TECHNIQUE: Lateral Recumbent Direct Myofascial Release

PROCEDURE: If the gluteus minimus is in spasm, there will be a tender lump just lateral to the upper one-third of the sacroiliac joint. With the pad of your thumb, first press slightly anteriorly and medially on the tightest point in this muscle. Maintain this balanced pressure until the release occurs and the muscle relaxes.

**Figure 4.23** Gluteus minimus technique

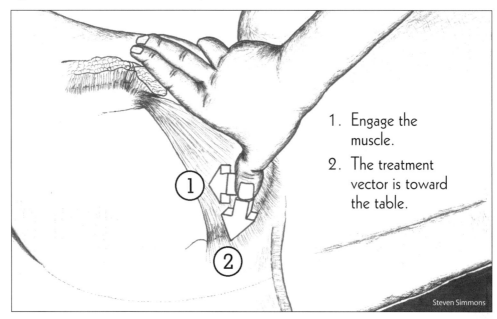

1. Engage the muscle.
2. The treatment vector is toward the table.

Steven Simmons

## Superior Gemellus

TECHNIQUE: Lateral recumbent direct myofascial release

PROCEDURE: Palpate for deep muscle spasm on a direct line halfway between the greater trochanter and the lower portion of the sacroiliac joint. With the pad of your thumb lying across the fibers of the middle of the superior gemellus muscle, maintain firm, steady pressure in a medial, anterior, and slightly inferior direction. Maintain this steady pressure until the muscle relaxes.

## Obturator Internus

TECHNIQUE: Lateral recumbent direct myofascial release

PROCEDURE: Moving inferiorly to the superior gemellus muscle, the next muscle that is encountered is the obturator internus. Move the pad of your thumb just inferior to the superior gemellus muscle, halfway between the greater trochanter and the inferior pole of the sacroiliac joint. If a spasm is found, maintain firm, steady pressure with the pad of your thumb perpendicular to the muscle fibers in a medial, anterior, and slightly inferior direction until the muscle relaxes.

## Inferior Gemellus

TECHNIQUE: Lateral recumbent direct myofascial release

PROCEDURE: Move the pad of your thumb even further in an inferior direction down the depression between the greater trochanter and the ischium, and palpate for spasm in the inferior gemellus muscle (halfway between the upper portion of the ischial tuberosity and the midportion of the greater trochanter). Treat with the pad of your thumb perpendicular to the fibers, maintaining firm, steady pressure anteriorly and medially.

## *Quadratus Femoris*

TECHNIQUE: Lateral recumbent direct myofascial release

PROCEDURE: Using the pad of your thumb, palpate the groove in which the sciatic nerve is found, halfway between the ischial tuberosity and the lesser trochanter. A muscle spasm at the lateral inferior portion of the buttocks indicates that the quadratus femoris muscle is involved. With the pad of your thumb perpendicular to the fibers, press in a superior, medial, and anterior direction. Maintain this balanced pressure until a release occurs.

**Figure 4.24** Quadratus femoris technique

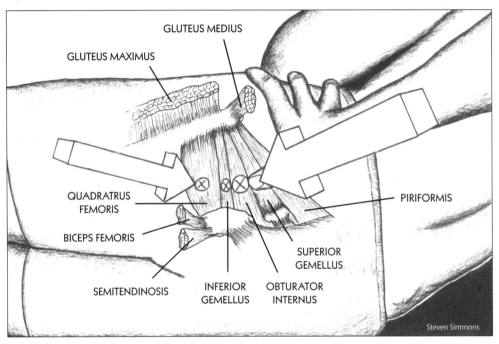

# *Piriformis*

TECHNIQUE: Lateral recumbent direct myofascial release

PROCEDURE: Locate spasms of the piriformis muscle very close to its point of insertion on the femur, slightly posterior and inferior to the superior portion of the greater trochanter. Maintain balanced firm pressure with the pad of your thumb medially (down toward the table) on this spasm until a release occurs.

**Figure 4.25**  Piriformis technique

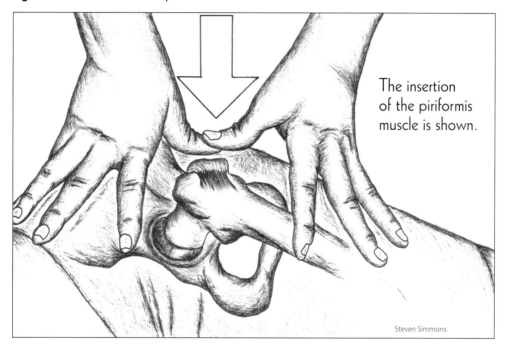

The insertion of the piriformis muscle is shown.

Steven Simmons

## *Gluteus Medius*

TECHNIQUE: Lateral Recumbent Direct Myofascial Release

PROCEDURE: The gluteus medius attaches to the superior portion of the greater trochanter. Locate the muscle spasm just superior to the greater trochanter of the femur. Using the pad of your thumb(s), maintain firm balanced pressure in a medial, slightly inferior, and slightly anterior direction close to the point of the hip. Maintain this steady balanced pressure until a release occurs. *Note:* treating all the previously described external hip rotators usually corrects sciatica.

**Figure 4.26** Gluteus medius technique

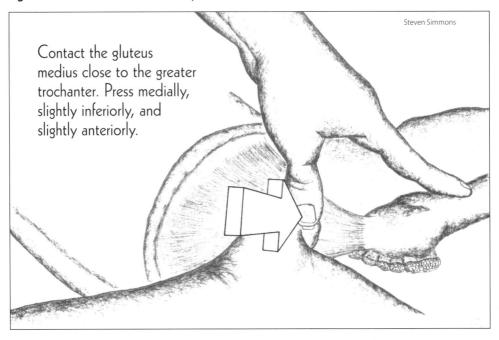

Contact the gluteus medius close to the greater trochanter. Press medially, slightly inferiorly, and slightly anteriorly.

Steven Simmons

**Figure 4.27** Gluteus medius hand placement

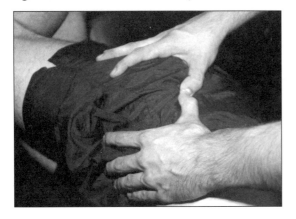

# Hip

## *Centering the Femur in the Acetabulum*

TECHNIQUE: Lateral recumbent indirect ligamentous articular release

SYMPTOMS/DIAGNOSIS: Hip pain, often due to a force transferred up from the lower extremity, or a fall directly on the hip

PATIENT: Lateral recumbent position with the hips and knees flexed. The affected hip is on top.

PHYSICIAN: Standing, facing the table behind the hip to be treated

PROCEDURE: Stabilize the ilium with the palm of your superior hand. With the greater trochanter centered in the palm of your inferior hand, generate a force directly down the neck of the femur to center the femoral head in the acetabulum. This involves a compression between your hands directed medially and slightly superiorly on the femur. Maintain this balanced force until the injury softens, and the tide begins to flow through the hip joint.

**Figure 4.28**  The femur in the acetabulum technique

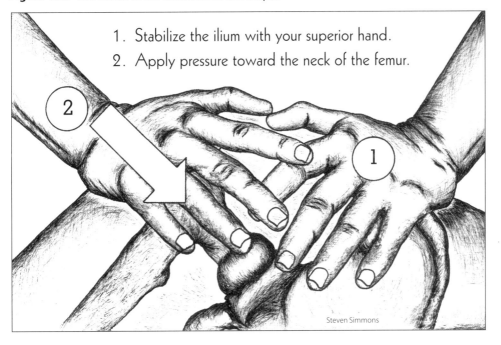

1. Stabilize the ilium with your superior hand.
2. Apply pressure toward the neck of the femur.

Steven Simmons

## *Second Hip Technique*

TECHNIQUE: Supine indirect ligamentous articular release

SYMPTOMS/DIAGNOSIS: Hip pain, often due to a force transferred up from the lower extremity, or a fall directly on the hip

PATIENT: Supine with the affected hip flexed 90° and the knee flexed. The other leg is straight.

PHYSICIAN: Standing at the side of the hip to be treated at the level of the knee, facing the head of the table

PROCEDURE: Roll the knee medially to raise the affected hip slightly off the table. Place the thenar eminence of your hand farthest from the table between the greater trochanter and the table, with your fingers pointing medially. Place the patient's knee in the depression just below your coricoid process to control the distal femur. Grasp the medial proximal aspect of the femur close to the femoral head with the middle finger, index finger, and thumb of your other hand. Use your shoulder to increase or decrease the

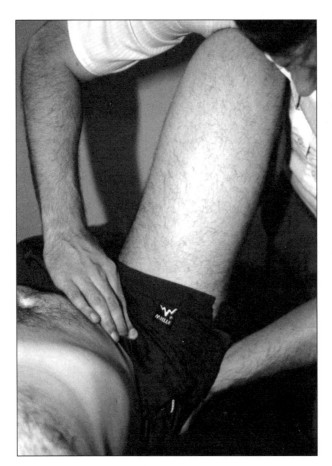

**Figure 4.29** Second hip technique hand placement

flexion at the hip and to slightly internally or externally rotate the femur. The patient's foot is dangling just off the table. Compress the hip slightly anteriorly and medially with your thenar eminence on the greater trochanter. With your medial hand grasping the femur close to the femoral head, generate pressure posteriorly and laterally with your middle finger, index finger, and thumb. Using your shoulder, locate the direction of balanced tension in the hip by slightly increasing or decreasing the flexion of the femur and slightly rotating the femur internally or externally. Balance the forces at the hip joint from all three contact points. When the release occurs, the connective tissue surrounding the head of the femur will readjust itself, all three vectors of force will melt, the femur will move back to its functional physiologic position, and the tide will begin flowing through the joint.

**Figure 4.30** Second hip technique

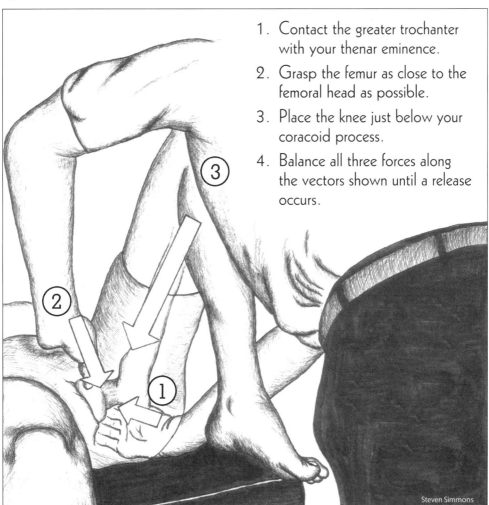

1. Contact the greater trochanter with your thenar eminence.

2. Grasp the femur as close to the femoral head as possible.

3. Place the knee just below your coracoid process.

4. Balance all three forces along the vectors shown until a release occurs.

Steven Simmons

# CHAPTER FIVE

# Pelvis and Lower Abdomen

# The Pelvis

## *Pelvic Diaphragm*

OUTER LAYER (Urogenital Diaphragm) and INNER LAYER (Pelvic Diaphragm)

The muscles and organs of the pelvic cavity connect with the endopelvic fascia. The endopelvic fascia in turn is connected to the medial umbilical ligaments, which connect to the umbilicus and the linea alba of the rectus sheath. Continuing superiorly from the umbilicus, the falciform ligaments and the round ligament of the liver, that is, the remnant of umbilical vein, attach to the liver as well as to the inferior surface of the diaphragm. Therefore, there is a direct anterior connection from the pelvic diaphragm to the respiratory diaphragm. The falciform ligament, round ligament, and the venous ligament run anterior to posterior and basically divide the liver into lobes. So, not only is there an inferior to superior connection from the pelvic diaphragm to the respiratory diaphragm, there is also an anterior to posterior connection of the anterior abdominal wall and posterior wall under the diaphragm.

The pelvic diaphragm is made up of two separate fascial planes. Since the pelvic diaphragm has two layers, the following procedure must first be performed on the outer layer, followed by the inner layer. The outer layer consists mainly of the superficial transverse perineal muscles and perineal membrane (inferior fascia of the urogenital diaphragm), and the inner layer consists mainly of the levator ani muscle. Only the levator ani intervenes between the ischiorectal fossa and the retropubic space.

The pelvic diaphragm acts like a physiologic diaphragm by helping pump fluid from the lower extremities into the abdominal cavity. When it is functioning properly, the pelvic diaphragm moves rhythmically with the "tide" and augments the flow of the tide through the pelvis. When it is dysfunctional, it inhibits the flow of the tide.

TECHNIQUE: Supine-Direct-Myofascial Release

SYMPTOMS/DIAGNOSIS: Urinary frequency, pain in the rectum, prostatitis, hemorrhoids, dyspareunia, or pain in the abdomen mimicking left ovarian pain

PATIENT: Supine, with the knees together and flexed to approximately 90° and the feet about a foot apart on the table

PHYSICIAN: Seated on the opposite side to be treated at midthigh level, facing the patient's head

PROCEDURE: Check both sides and then treat the one that is tense, not the one that is lax. Using your right hand to treat the left pelvic diaphragm (or your left hand to treat the right pelvic diaphragm), work on the far side of the pelvis. To engage the diaphragm, follow the natural curve of the medial surface of the far ischial tuberosity, pressing superiorly and laterally with the tip of your thumb. If a firm barrier is met, that layer of the pelvic diaphragm is in spasm. Maintain a steady balanced pressure until a release occurs and that layer softens.

When the outer layer has released, be sure to treat the inner layer by continuing to press in a more superior and lateral direction until a second barrier is felt. Maintain a firm balanced tension until a second release occurs.

In our experience, the left pelvic diaphragm appears to be more dysfunctional than the right. Also note that if both sides are tight, treating the tighter side often releases the other side.

**Figure 5.1** Pelvic diaphragm technique

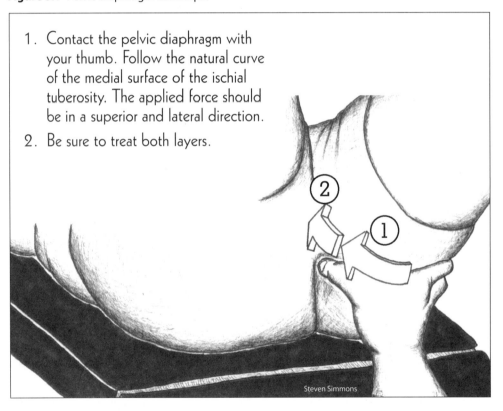

1. Contact the pelvic diaphragm with your thumb. Follow the natural curve of the medial surface of the ischial tuberosity. The applied force should be in a superior and lateral direction.

2. Be sure to treat both layers.

Steven Simmons

**Figure 5.2** Pelvic diaphragm release hand placement. Note that the thumb is on the inside of the thigh so that the patient is more comfortable, and the fingertips are grasping the outside of the thigh.

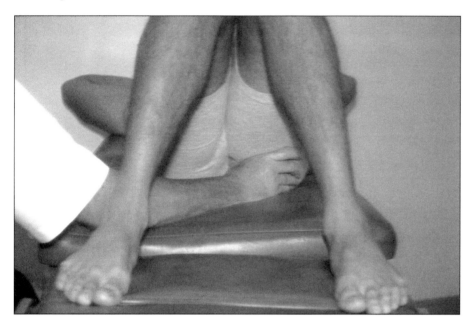

## *Presacral Fascia*

TECHNIQUE: Supine direct myofascial release

SYMPTOMS/DIAGNOSIS: Pelvic pain, sacral restriction, low back pain, testicular swelling or hydroceles

PATIENT: Supine

PHYSICIAN: Standing, facing the side of the table at the level of the pelvis

PROCEDURE: The presacral fascia extends down the anterior surface of the sacrum as a continuation of the prevertebral fascia and attaches to the anterior surface of vertebra S2. You are effecting a change in the presacral fascia by means of the medial umbilical ligaments, which attach to the presacral fascia. You will notice from the effect that this technique has on testicular swelling that you are also affecting strains in the inguinal rings.

Form a horseshoe with your thumb and the middle finger of your dominant hand contacting the medial umbilical ligaments at approximately the level of the deep inguinal rings. These are located about two inches above the pubes and about two inches from the midline. Press posteriorly and slightly inferiorly, maintaining a balanced tension until the release occurs. When it does, you should feel a caudad and cephalad pivoting motion. This motion follows the internal curve of the sacrum.

**Figure 5.3** Presacral fascia technique

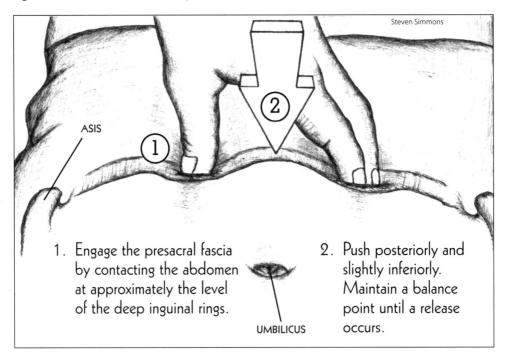

Steven Simmons

ASIS

① ②

1. Engage the presacral fascia by contacting the abdomen at approximately the level of the deep inguinal rings.

UMBILICUS

2. Push posteriorly and slightly inferiorly. Maintain a balance point until a release occurs.

**Figure 5.4** Presacral fascia technique: lateral view

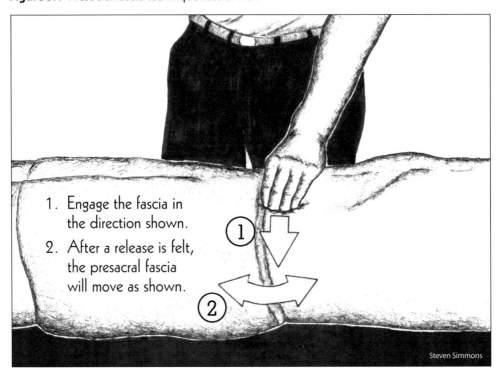

1. Engage the fascia in the direction shown.
2. After a release is felt, the presacral fascia will move as shown.

①

②

Steven Simmons

# Sacroiliac Release Techniques

The following are two different sacroiliac release techniques. When the patient has a lateral compression problem in the sacroiliac joint, you will usually encounter a great deal of resistance in the tissue when using the first technique, decompression sacral release. The second technique, cross-hand sacral release, will treat this compression dysfunction more efficiently.

## *Decompression Sacral Release*

TECHNIQUE: Supine direct ligamentous articular release

SYMPTOMS/DIAGNOSIS: Sacroiliac pain, low back pain, "hip" pain, or pain down the legs

PATIENT: Supine with the knees and hips bent so that the knees are together and the feet flat on the table, approximately one foot apart

PHYSICIAN: Sitting at the side of the table at the level of the patient's thigh, facing the patient's head

PROCEDURE: Have the patient raise their buttocks off the table so you can place your hands under the patient. Your dominant hand should be under the far sacroiliac joint. Your nondominant hand should be under the near sacroiliac joint. For example, if you are right-handed you will sit to the patient's right and put your right hand under their left sacroiliac joint. Line up your

**Figure 5.5** Decompression sacral release

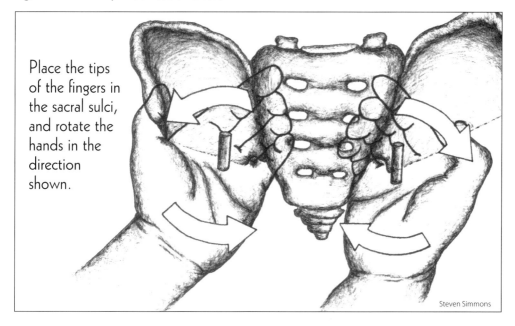

Place the tips of the fingers in the sacral sulci, and rotate the hands in the direction shown.

Steven Simmons

fingertips in the sacral sulcus on each side. The thenar eminences of each hand should contact the inferior gemellus muscle on each side. Have the patient lower their entire weight onto your hands keeping their knees bent. Imagine an axis perpendicular to the table passing through the palms of each hand. Rotate your fingers laterally and your thenar eminences medially around this axis, drawing the iliae laterally and inferiorly off of the sacrum. Maintain this balanced tension until a release is felt, and the sacrum is free to move normally.

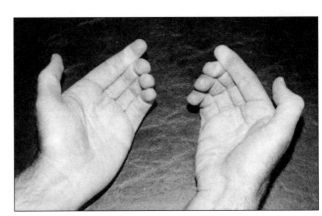

**Figure 5.6**
Hand position for the decompression sacral release

## *Cross-Hand Sacral Release*

TECHNIQUE: Supine indirect ligamentous articular release

SYMPTOMS/DIAGNOSIS: Sacroiliac pain, low back pain, hip pain, or pain down the legs

PATIENT: Supine

PHYSICIAN: Sitting at the patient's right side, facing the patient's head. (If you are left-handed, switch sides.)

PROCEDURE: Slide your right hand under the patient and grasp the patient's sacrum. Your fingertips will be at the level of the sacral base and the coccyx will be in the proximal portion of your palm. Using your left hand, bridge the posterior superior iliac spines with your fingertips contacting the left posterior superior iliac spine, and your thenar eminence contacting the right posterior superior iliac spine. Compress the posterior superior iliac spines together with your left hand. With your right hand, push slightly anteriorly on the sacrum to disengage it, and then carry it superiorly to a balance point with the two contact points of your left hand on the two posterior superior iliac spines—like putting equal pressure on the feet of a tripod. Maintain all three points of contact—both posterior superior iliac spines and the sacral base—at a balance point until a release occurs. When this happens, you will feel the forces opposing your compression soften, and the sacrum will be free to move.

**Figure 5.7** Cross-hand sacral release

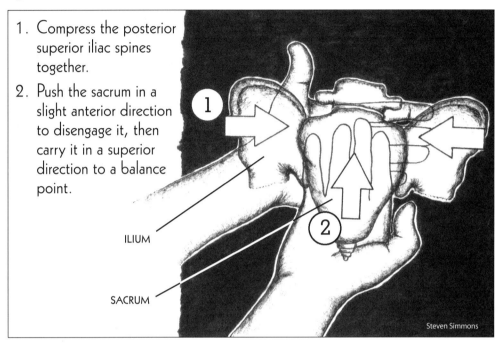

1. Compress the posterior superior iliac spines together.

2. Push the sacrum in a slight anterior direction to disengage it, then carry it in a superior direction to a balance point.

ILIUM

SACRUM

Steven Simmons

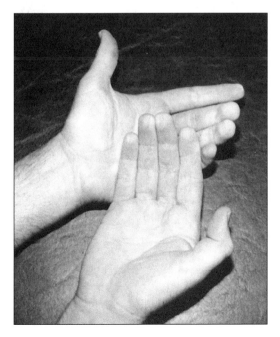

**Figure 5.8** Hand position for cross-hand sacral release

## *Pelvic Torsion Technique*

Torsions of the pelvis are maintained by superior and inferior subluxations at the pubic symphysis. The side with the superior subluxation will have an apparent short leg.

TECHNIQUE: Supine indirect ligamentous articular release

SYMPTOMS/DIAGNOSIS: Groin or pubic pain, apparent leg length difference, or pelvic torsions

PATIENT: Supine

PHYSICIAN: Standing at the side of the table at the level of the mid-thigh, facing the patient's head

PROCEDURE: Contact both anterior superior iliac spines with your hands, cupping them in your palms. Compress the spines together to disengage the posterior aspect of the pubic symphysis. Determine in which direction the innominates move more easily by first rotating one side anteriorly and the other side posteriorly, then reversing directions. To treat, rotate the innominates in the direction of least resistance, and maintain a balanced tension until a release occurs. The innominates will rotate a little past their "zero points" when they release. Once the release has occurred, slowly decrease the rotational pressure and allow the innominates to return to their normal position. They will then start rotating internally and externally with the tide.

**Figure 5.9**  Pelvic torsion technique

1. Cup the anterior superior iliac spines in your palms and compress them together.

2. Rotate the ilia in the direction of least resistance until a release is felt.

Steven Simmons

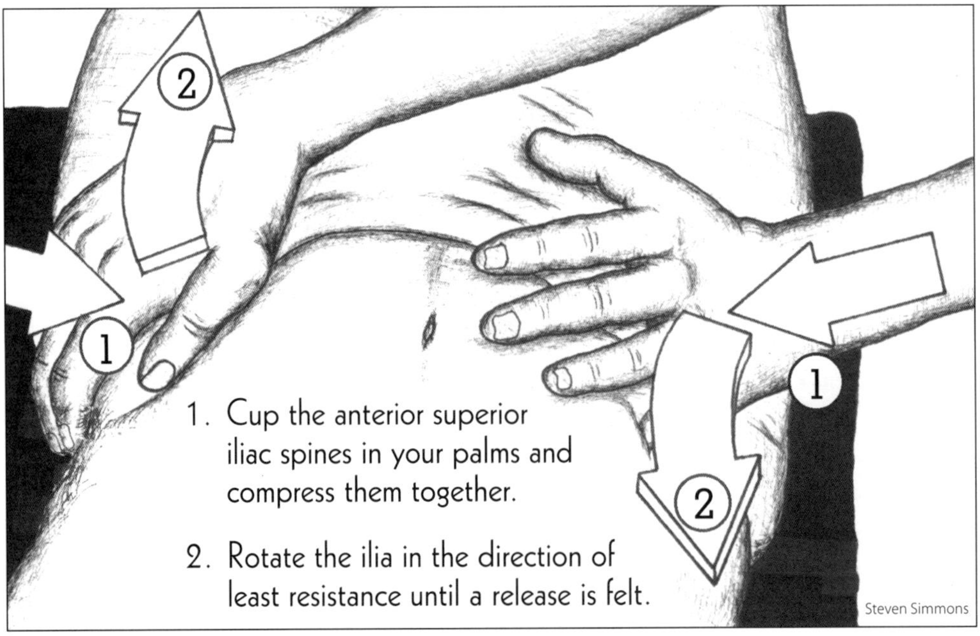

# Lower Abdomen

## *Inguinal Ligament*

TECHNIQUE: Supine direct ligamentous articular release

SYMPTOMS/DIAGNOSIS: Pain in the groin, meralgia parastheticia (that is, pain or numbness in the anterior thigh), or the knee collapses on standing up from a seated position. The latter is due to dysfunction of the quadriceps. A torsion in the pelvis can result in an inguinal ligament dysfunction. A tight inguinal ligament will impinge on the femoral nerve, artery, and vein. This may result in quadriceps weakness and a complaint of the knee collapsing out from under the patient. Impingement of the lateral femoral cutaneous nerve may cause meralgia parestheticia (also known as Bernhardt-Roth syndrome). Pain or numbness may also be present on the anterior or medial thigh.

PATIENT: Supine

PHYSICIAN: Standing at the level of the mid-thigh on the side to be treated, facing the head of the table

PROCEDURE: Contact the middle of the inguinal ligament with your hypothenar eminence and press in a superior, medial, and posterior direction perpendicular to the ligament. Maintain steady balanced pressure until a release occurs and the tight ligament softens.

**Figure 5.10**  Inguinal ligament technique

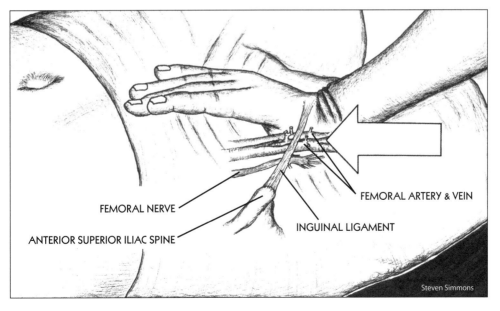

FEMORAL ARTERY & VEIN

FEMORAL NERVE

INGUINAL LIGAMENT

ANTERIOR SUPERIOR ILIAC SPINE

Steven Simmons

## *Iliopsoas Muscle*

TECHNIQUE: Supine direct myofascial release

SYMPTOMS/DIAGNOSIS: If bilateral iliopsoas spasm is present, the patient will be bent forward at the waist when standing. If unilateral iliopsoas spasm is present, the patient will be bent forward and leaning toward the affected side when standing. If the patient attempts to stand straight, the side of the pelvis with the iliopsoas spasm will be higher than the other. The iliopsoas muscle spasm keeps the hip flexed whether the patient is standing or supine. The patient pushes on his thighs to stand up from a seated position.

PATIENT: Supine

PHYSICIAN: Standing, facing the table at the level of the pelvis opposite the side to be treated

PROCEDURE: Using the distal pad of the thumb of your dominant hand, contact the iliopsoas muscle lateral to the femoral artery and just inferior and medial to the anterior superior iliac spine. Reinforce your pressure by placing the thumb of your other hand on top. Engage the muscle initially by directing a force posteriorly, toward the table, on the medial aspect of the muscle. Once the muscle is engaged, carry a steady, balanced force laterally until a release is felt and the muscle relaxes.

**Figure 5.11** Iliopsoas technique

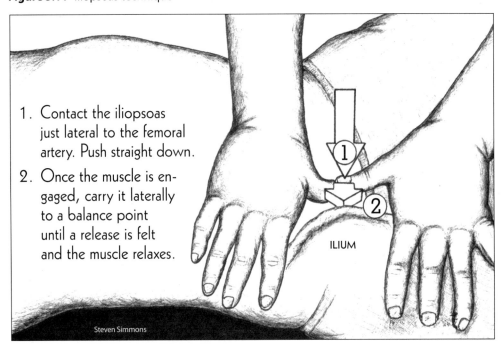

1. Contact the iliopsoas just lateral to the femoral artery. Push straight down.

2. Once the muscle is engaged, carry it laterally to a balance point until a release is felt and the muscle relaxes.

ILIUM

Steven Simmons

## *Iliolumbar Ligaments and Erector Spinae Muscles*

The following technique is an often-overlooked pearl which can greatly enhance your results in sacral and lumbar treatments. When you release the iliolumbar ligament, continue to move anteriorly and superiorly to release the latissimus dorsi (as described in Chapter 6).

TECHNIQUE: Lateral recumbent direct ligamentous articular release

SYMPTOMS/DIAGNOSIS: Pain in lower back, radicular pain down the back of the leg, or restricted motion of the sacroiliac joints and lumbar spine

PATIENT: Lateral recumbent position with the knees and hips flexed, injured side up

PHYSICIAN: Standing at the side of the table behind the patient at the level of the mid- to lower thorax, facing the patient's feet

PROCEDURE: With the pad of the thumb of your hand closest to the patient, contact the iliolumbar ligament just medial and slightly superior to the posterior superior iliac spine between the ilium and the vertebrae L4–L5. Press anteriorly to contact the iliolumbar ligaments. If they are strained, they will feel like a firm barrier. Secondarily, press anteriorly and inferiorly with your thumb, maintaining balanced pressure at this barrier until a release occurs. The erector spinae muscles relax when the strained iliolumbar ligaments release. Treating the strained iliolumbar ligaments is essential to achieving a full release of the sacrum and lumbar spine.

**Figure 5.12**  Erector spinae and iliolumbar ligament technique

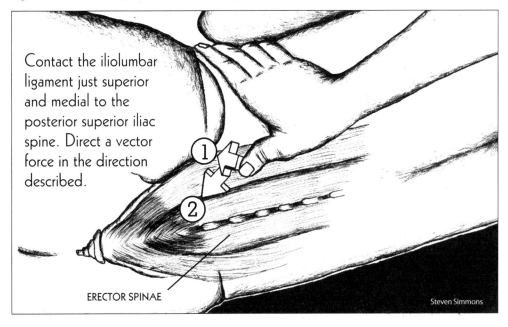

# CHAPTER SIX

# Abdomen and Thorax

# Abdomen

## *Median Umbilical Ligament*

The median umbilical ligament is the remnant of the prenatal urachus, a canal in the fetus that connects the bladder with the allantois. After birth this structure is part of the connection between the pelvic fascia and the diaphragm.

TECHNIQUE: Supine direct myofascial release

SYMPTOMS/DIAGNOSIS: Pain in suprapubic area or urinary frequency

PATIENT: Supine

PHYSICIAN: Standing, facing the table at the level of the median umbilical ligament

PROCEDURE: With the hands and fingers perpendicular to the abdomen, line up the fingertips along the linea alba halfway between the pubic symphysis and the umbilicus. With flat hands, straight fingers, and the fingertips of the index and middle fingers of each hand touching their counterparts, press the ulnar aspects of the fingertips directly into the midline. Press posteriorly (directly down toward the table) until resistance is met. Maintain steady pressure against this barrier until it begins to "melt," then rotate the upper portions of your hands closer together and spread your fingertips apart. Once your fingertips are fully spread apart, the treatment is complete.

**Figure 6.1** Median umbilical ligament technique

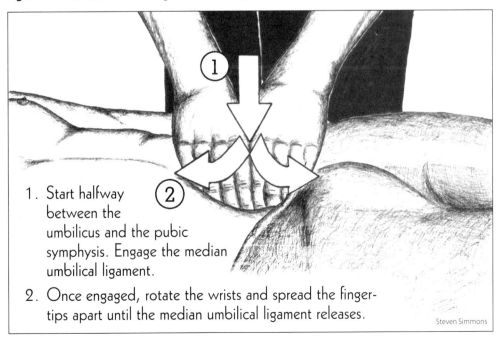

1. Start halfway between the umbilicus and the pubic symphysis. Engage the median umbilical ligament.

2. Once engaged, rotate the wrists and spread the fingertips apart until the median umbilical ligament releases.

Steven Simmons

## *Umbilicus*

TECHNIQUE: Supine indirect myofascial release

SYMPTOMS/DIAGNOSIS: Abdominal pain, asthma, pelvic pain, and gastrointestinal complaints

PATIENT: Supine

PHYSICIAN: Standing, facing the table slightly inferior to the umbilicus

PROCEDURE: Inspect the umbilicus for folds along its rim. (A smooth, rounded contour is normal.) Use the pad of your thumb to make contact with the umbilicus. Press deep enough to disengage the umbilicus, then rotate the thumb clockwise and counterclockwise to determine in which direction it most easily moves. Rotate steadily in the direction of least resistance until your thumb has turned a full 360°. It helps to stand on the patient's right to go clockwise and on the patient's left to go counterclockwise. When a barrier is met, maintain steady, balanced pressure against the resistance until a release is felt. Slowly remove your thumb from on top of the umbilicus and inspect to see whether the fold or folds have decreased or disappeared.

**Figure 6.2** Umbilicus technique

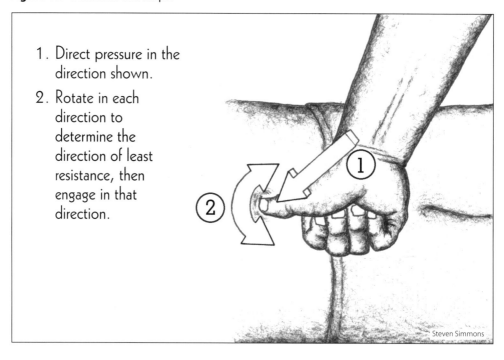

1. Direct pressure in the direction shown.

2. Rotate in each direction to determine the direction of least resistance, then engage in that direction.

Steven Simmons

## *Superior Linea Alba*

TECHNIQUE: Supine direct myofascial release

SYMPTOMS/DIAGNOSIS: Pain in the epigastric area, indigestion, or shock[1]

PATIENT: Supine

PHYSICIAN: Standing, facing the table at the level of the epigastric area

PROCEDURE: With your hands and fingers perpendicular to the abdomen, line up your fingertips along the linea alba midway between the xyphoid and umbilicus. With straight fingers and hands and with the fingertips of your index and middle fingers touching their counterparts, press your distal lateral fingertips directly into the midline. Press posteriorly (directly down toward the table) until resistance is met. Maintain steady pressure against this barrier until you feel a release, then rotate the upper portions of your hands closer together and spread your fingertips apart. Once your fingertips are fully spread apart, the treatment is complete.

**Figure 6.3** Superior linea alba technique

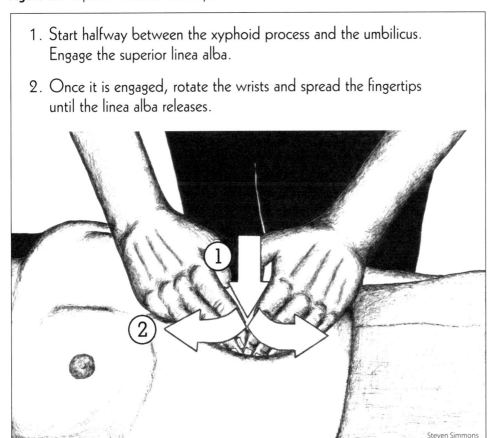

1. Start halfway between the xyphoid process and the umbilicus. Engage the superior linea alba.

2. Once it is engaged, rotate the wrists and spread the fingertips until the linea alba releases.

Steven Simmons

## *Falciform Ligament*

TECHNIQUE: Supine direct myofascial release

SYMPTOMS/DIAGNOSIS: Pain in upper right quadrant of the abdomen

PATIENT: Supine

PHYSICIAN: Standing, facing the table on the patient's left just inferior to the diaphragm

PROCEDURE: To locate the falciform ligament, place the pad of your thumb parallel to the right lower costal margin, approximately one-half to one inch below the xyphoid process, and just to the right of the midline. Press with balanced tension across the falciform ligament using the pad of your thumb. (The falciform ligament lies approximately halfway between the midaxillary line and tip of the xyphoid process along the edge of the rib cage on the right.) Press in a posterior and superior direction. Test for ease of motion along the costal margin; this is usually in the lateral direction. Maintain balanced pressure across the falciform ligament with the pad of your thumb until a release occurs and the tension in the ligament dissipates. You will no longer be able to palpate the falciform ligament.

**Figure 6.4** Falciform ligament technique

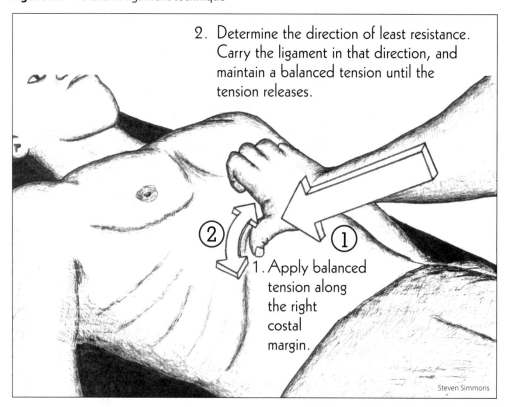

2. Determine the direction of least resistance. Carry the ligament in that direction, and maintain a balanced tension until the tension releases.

1. Apply balanced tension along the right costal margin.

Steven Simmons

## *Coronary Ligament*

TECHNIQUE: Supine direct myofascial release

SYMPTOMS/DIAGNOSIS: Pain in the upper left quadrant of the abdomen

PATIENT: Supine

PHYSICIAN: Standing, facing the table on the right side of the patient just inferior to the diaphragm

PROCEDURE: The coronary ligament is contacted through the extraperitoneal fascia and the abdominal peritoneum just below the left costal margin, which then runs up under the respiratory diaphragm and reflects back over the liver as the coronary ligament. The contact must be made through the skin, subcutaneous fascia, and abdominal muscles until the extraperitoneal fascia and peritoneum are contacted. (Pressure can be in the 10- to 20-pound range.) The coronary ligament is treated via these tissues.[2] Place the pad of your thumb just below the left costal margin and press with balanced tension across the tight tissue you feel there in a posterior, lateral, and superior direction until a release occurs. When this happens, all the tension in this off-shoot of the coronary ligament dissipates and you will no longer be able to feel this tension.

**Figure 6.5** Coronary ligament technique

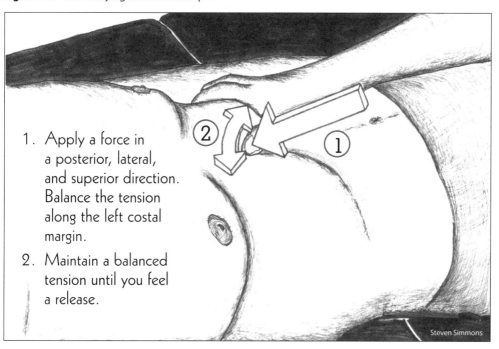

1. Apply a force in a posterior, lateral, and superior direction. Balance the tension along the left costal margin.

2. Maintain a balanced tension until you feel a release.

Steven Simmons

## *Latissimus Dorsi*

When you release the iliolumbar ligament as described in Chapter 5, continue to move anteriorly and superiorly to release the latissimus dorsi. As noted in Chapter 5, this technique commonly follows the treatment of the iliolumbar ligament.

TECHNIQUE: Lateral recumbent direct myofascial release

SYMPTOMS/DIAGNOSIS: Pain in the posterior lateral lower back or restricted motion of the shoulder

PATIENT: Lateral recumbent position with the knees and hips flexed, affected side up

PHYSICIAN: Standing behind the patient at the level of the shoulder blade, facing the patient's feet

PROCEDURE: With the pad of the thumb of your hand closest to the patient, contact the origin of the latissimus dorsi along and superior to the posterior lateral iliac crest. Maintain balanced steady pressure directed anteriorly, medially, and inferiorly at this point until a release occurs. Maintaining this steady pressure, follow the iliac crest anteriorly to make sure that the entire muscle has released.

**Figure 6.6** Latissimus dorsi technique

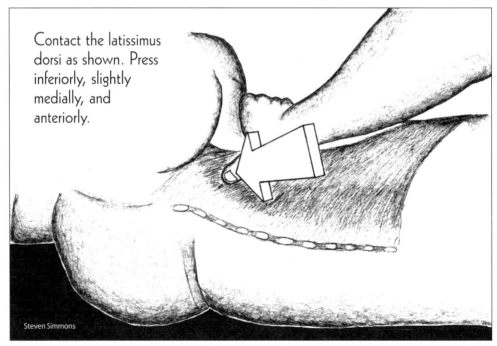

Contact the latissimus dorsi as shown. Press inferiorly, slightly medially, and anteriorly.

Steven Simmons

## *Internal and External Abdominal Oblique Muscles*

TECHNIQUE: Lateral recumbent direct myofascial release

SYMPTOMS/DIAGNOSIS: Lateral abdominal pain or restricted rotational motion of lumbar and lower thoracic spine

PATIENT: Lateral recumbent position with the knees and hips flexed, injured side up

PHYSICIAN: Standing, facing the table, behind the patient at the level of the iliac crest

PROCEDURE: Using the pad of the thumb of your dominant hand reinforced with your other hand, contact the lateral abdominal wall halfway between the iliac crest and the lower costal margin. Maintain balanced pressure medially and slightly inferiorly until a release occurs and your thumbs sink deeper into the abdomen.

**Figure 6.7** Internal and external abdominal oblique muscles technique

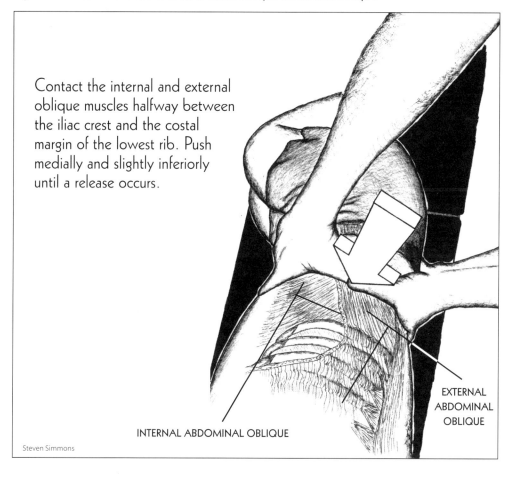

Contact the internal and external oblique muscles halfway between the iliac crest and the costal margin of the lowest rib. Push medially and slightly inferiorly until a release occurs.

EXTERNAL ABDOMINAL OBLIQUE

INTERNAL ABDOMINAL OBLIQUE

Steven Simmons

# Thorax

## *Lower Ribs and Respiratory Diaphragm*

TECHNIQUE: Supine indirect ligamentous articular release

SYMPTOMS/DIAGNOSIS: Lower chest pain, difficulty drawing deep breath, or flaring of the lower ribs

PATIENT: Supine

PHYSICIAN: Standing or seated at the side of the table, facing the patient's head slightly inferior to the diaphragm

PROCEDURE: Grasp across the lower ribs with the palms and fingers of both hands. Press your two hands toward the xyphoid process, maintaining a balanced tension between your hands. The compression should not be crushing, but likewise it should be more than just touching the skin. The pressure varies depending on how much tension is present in the ribs, usually five to ten pounds. Maintain this balanced pressure until the resistance releases and the hands compress more deeply toward each other. Slowly release the pressure as soon as the resistance lessens until the ribs are fully expanded. This procedure also helps release the diaphragm.

**Figure 6.8** Lateral compression for the lower ribs and respiratory diaphragm

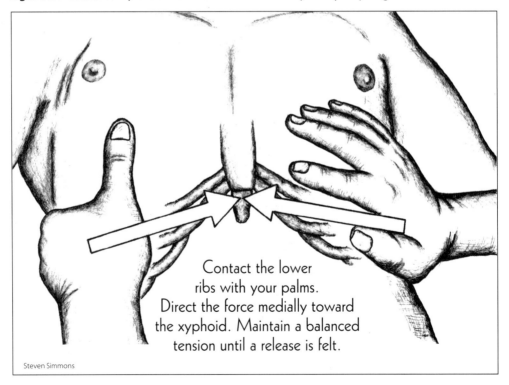

Contact the lower ribs with your palms. Direct the force medially toward the xyphoid. Maintain a balanced tension until a release is felt.

Steven Simmons

# *Respiratory Diaphragm*

TECHNIQUE: Supine direct myofascial release

SYMPTOMS/DIAGNOSIS: Inability to take a deep breath

PATIENT: Supine

PHYSICIAN: Standing at the side of the table, facing the patient's head at approximately the level of the pelvis

PROCEDURE: Using the heel of your dominant hand, scoop up the viscera, starting from just above the umbilicus. Be careful not to traumatize the aorta. Compress the viscera in a superior direction toward the lower chest, causing the upper portion of the respiratory diaphragm to move superiorly and assume a nice dome shape. Maintain firm, balanced pressure until the respiratory diaphragm relaxes. This procedure also moves any lymphatic fluid trapped below the diaphragm in the cisterna chyli up across the diaphragm and into the thoracic duct.

Also, if needed, you can treat the midthoracic spine at the same time by grasping across the thoracic paravertebral muscles in the area of the dysfunction with your nondominant hand and maintaining pressure between your two hands. If this is done, the procedure is complete when you feel the thoracic dysfunction relax in your nondominant hand, and the "balloon" collapse in the palm of your dominant hand.

**Figure 6.9** Respiratory diaphragm technique

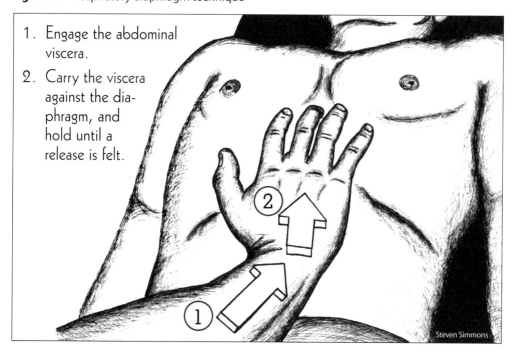

1. Engage the abdominal viscera.
2. Carry the viscera against the diaphragm, and hold until a release is felt.

Steven Simmons

## *Sternum*

TECHNIQUE: Supine indirect ligamentous articular release

SYMPTOMS/DIAGNOSIS: Anterior midchest pain

PATIENT: Supine

PHYSICIAN: Standing at the head of the table, facing the patient's feet

PROCEDURE: Place the heel of your dominant hand on the manubrium, and grasp the body of the sternum just above the xyphoid process (the xyphosternal junction) with the pads of your fingers. Press the manubrium posteriorly and inferiorly. Contract your hand slightly to increase the flexion at the angle of Louis. If necessary, reinforce the compression with your other hand by placing it over the dorsum of the treating hand. Now that you have the sternum disengaged, see if it tips left or right. If it does tip, slightly exaggerate the tip in that direction, and maintain the tip as you try rotating the sternum clockwise and counterclockwise. Rotate in the direction of least resistance. Maintain all these vectors of force until the release occurs. The sternum should rotate back to midline, level from side to side, and flex or extend as needed to return to its normal physiologic position. Once the release has occurred, the sternum will start flexing and extending with the "tide."

**Figure 6.10** Sternum technique

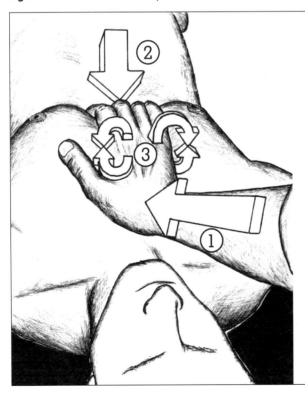

1. Contact the sternum with the heel of your hand on the manubrium and with the fingertips at the xyphosternal junction. Press in the direction shown.

2. Compress the sternum between the heel of your hand and your fingertips by flexing your hand.

3. Balance the sternum in the directions shown.

Steven Simmons

## *Pectus Excavatum*

TECHNIQUE: Supine indirect ligamentous articular release

SYMPTOMS/DIAGNOSIS: Concave sternum

PATIENT: Supine

PHYSICIAN: Standing at the head of the table, facing the patient's feet

PROCEDURE: The treatment of the pectus excavatum is the same as described above for the sternum except that the concavity of the sternum is exaggerated by carrying your fingertips more posteriorly and inferiorly. Repeat at one- to two-month intervals until the condition diminishes or is resolved.

## *Pectus Carinatum*

TECHNIQUE: Supine indirect ligamentous articular release

SYMPTOMS/DIAGNOSIS: Pigeon breasted

PATIENT: Supine

PHYSICIAN: Seated at the side of the table, facing the patient's head

PROCEDURE: Place the palms of your hands on the sides of the chest with the fingers of your far hand pointed posteriorly and the fingers of your near hand pointed anteriorly. With the palms of your hands, compress the middle to upper ribs together, which exaggerates the protruding sternum. Come to a firm balance point between your two hands. Maintain pressure until a release occurs and your hands move toward each other. Allow the chest to expand as you slowly remove your hands. Repeat at one to two month intervals until the condition diminishes or is resolved.

# Somatoemotional Releases

In our experience, the sternum and the anterior cervical fascia are the most common areas for somatoemotional releases. There must have been a strong emotion associated with the injury for this to occur. For example, if the patient is injured from striking a tree after skidding on an icy road, a somatoemotional release will probably not occur. However, if the patient is injured in exactly the same accident but another passenger is killed, then a somatoemotional release will probably occur at the moment the injury to the sternum is resolved.

## Restricted Middle Rib Group
### *Bucket-Handle Motion of the Middle Ribs*

TECHNIQUE: Lateral recumbent direct ligamentous articular release

SYMPTOMS/DIAGNOSIS: Lateral chest pain, pain inside the shoulder blades, costochondritis, rigid chest, or mechanical restriction to breathing[3]

PATIENT: Lateral recumbent position with the injured ribs up

PHYSICIAN: Standing, facing the table behind the patient just inferior to the axilla

PROCEDURE: Using the palms of your hands, compress ribs 4 through 8 directly toward the table. Maintain firm, balanced pressure until both the rigidity dissipates and the ribs start moving normally in their bucket-handle motion during respiration.

**Figure 6.11** Restricted middle rib group technique

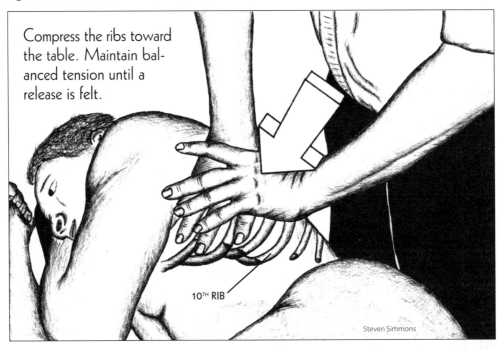

## *Ribs 2 through 12*

TECHNIQUE: Supine indirect ligamentous articular release

SYMPTOMS/DIAGNOSIS: Pain between the shoulder blades, pain lateral to the thoracic spine, costochondritis, or chest pain, especially on twisting or turning

PATIENT: Supine

PHYSICIAN: Seated facing the table slightly superior to and on the same side of the rib to be treated

PROCEDURE: Slide your supine hand under the patient's thorax. Grasp the angle of the dysfunctional rib with your finger pads (usually the index, middle, and ring fingers) and carry it anteriorly to disengage it, then superiorly and laterally. Maintain balanced traction until the rib releases. When the release occurs, the rib moves superiorly, sweeps laterally, and then drops inferiorly into its socket.

**Figure 6.12**  Supine lower ribs 2 through 12 technique

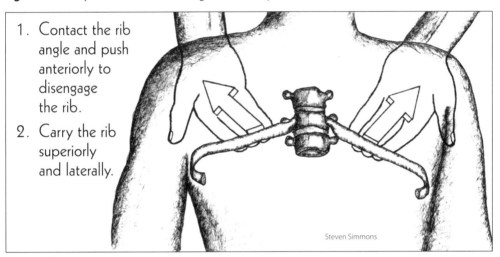

1. Contact the rib angle and push anteriorly to disengage the rib.
2. Carry the rib superiorly and laterally.

Steven Simmons

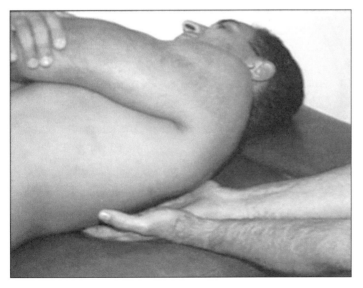

**Figure 6.13**  Supine lower ribs 2 through 12 hand placement. In the photo the patient is turned on his side so you can see the hand placement. For the treatment, however, the patient is supine.

## *Second and Third Ribs (Lateral Recumbent)*[4]

TECHNIQUE: Lateral recumbent indirect ligamentous articular release

SYMPTOMS/DIAGNOSIS: Pain medial to the upper shoulder blade or costochondritis of the upper ribs

PATIENT: Lateral recumbent position with the injured rib(s) up

PHYSICIAN: Standing at the side of the table behind patient at approximately the level of the diaphragm, and angling toward the head

PROCEDURE: Grasp the injured rib adjacent to the sternum with the fingertips of one hand. With the fingertips of your other hand, grasp the angle of the same rib adjacent to the spine. Push anteriorly on the angle of the rib to disengage the rib, and carry the rib head superiorly and laterally. Compress medially and slightly superiorly with both thumbs at the lateral aspect of the same rib. (On the second and third ribs, your thumbs will be in the axilla.) Bring all three contact points—the lateral aspect of the rib and the anterior and posterior ends of the rib—into balance until the rib releases and returns to a normal physiologic position. At this point, the rib(s) should start moving with respiration.

**Figure 6.14** Upper ribs treated in the lateral recumbent position

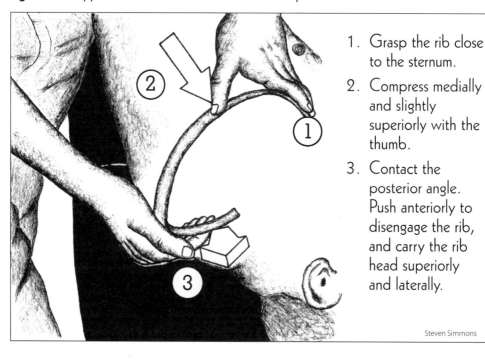

1. Grasp the rib close to the sternum.

2. Compress medially and slightly superiorly with the thumb.

3. Contact the posterior angle. Push anteriorly to disengage the rib, and carry the rib head superiorly and laterally.

Steven Simmons

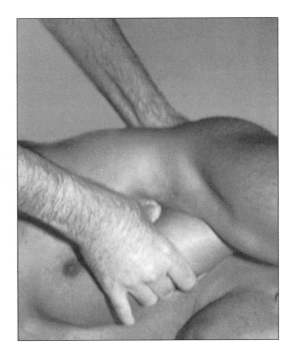

**Figure 6.15** Lateral recumbent upper ribs hand placement

## *First Rib (Elevated)*

If the first rib is dysfunctional, it will usually be pulled superiorly out of its socket and a lump will be found on that side just anterior to the trapezius at the lateral aspect of the junction of the cervical and thoracic spine. If both first ribs are pulled up, you will find a lump on both sides.

TECHNIQUE: Supine direct ligamentous articular release

SYMPTOMS/DIAGNOSIS: Pain at the base of the neck, restricted rotation of the neck to the affected side, numbness of the ring finger and fifth finger on the affected side, headaches, or pain behind the eye on the affected side

PATIENT: Supine

PHYSICIAN: Seated at the head of the table, facing the patient's feet

PROCEDURE: Run the pads of your thumbs inferiorly along the lateral aspect of the cervical vertebrae until you contact the superior surface of the first rib, which will feel like a hard lump adjacent to the spine. Press directly inferiorly (toward the patient's feet) on the superior surface of the head of the first rib.[5] Using the pad of your thumb, maintain this steady, firm, balanced pressure inferiorly until a release occurs and the rib slips back down into its socket between the vertebra. The lump will disappear.

Balance is especially critical in the area of the thoracic outlet. There is a delicate level of pressure that the patient will tolerate, and this is the balance point. If you exceed this level, the patient will not tolerate the pain, and guarding will hinder the treatment. "Balance" is not cramming beyond the tissue's elastic limits, and yet it requires a certain amount of force. Enough pressure is applied to accomplish a release. The key to successful treatment of any part of the body is this delicate balance.

**Figure 6.16** Elevated first rib technique

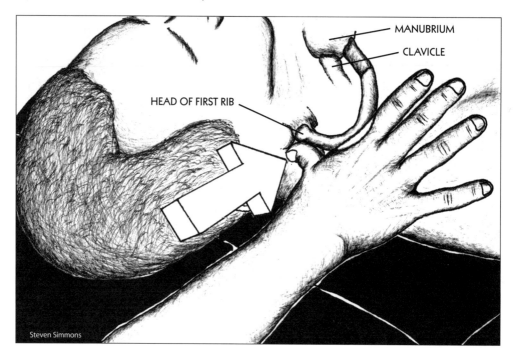

1   This was one of the main techniques used by Robert Fulford, D.O., to rid the body of the effects of shock.

2   The use of adjacent tissue to achieve an affect holds true for other techniques as well, for example, the presacral fascia (which uses the medial umbilical ligament and fold).

3   This treatment is necessary if, when medially compressed, the lateral ribs feel very rigid and have impaired bucket-handle motion, that is, the movement of the lateral portion of the ribs superiorly and inferiorly with respiration.

4   The Dallas Osteopathic Study Group developed this technique to relieve the strain on physicians that can occur when treating these ribs with the patient in a seated position as attributed to Sutherland in the Lippincott article. This procedure can also be used for any injured rib(s).

5   This is a direct technique.

# CHAPTER SEVEN

# Spinal Column

When treating the spine, remember that you are treating structures derived from the embryonic axial core and, importantly, keep a mental image of the planes of the somites that formed the sclerotomes within which the vertebrae developed. This imaging process is similar to the one used by plastic surgeons who maintain a mental image of the dermatomes in order to minimize the resulting scars.

During development, the sclerotomes shift from their embryonic transverse plane to a diagonal plane, angling from their posterior margin superiorly to their anterior margin. In other words, they are like a stack of washers that shift such that their anterior margin moves superiorly. This shifting of the planes of the sclerotomes occurs when the infant straightens out from a tight C-curl to a gentle double S-curve. The facets form along these functional planes. The difference in the angles of the facets in the three regions of the spine is also dictated by the somites from which the regional vertebrae were derived. Interesting embryological research in recent years seems to confirm this clinical impression.

> Somites produce verterbrae characteristic of specific regions and segments of the trunk.
>
> While somites throughout the trunk are morphologically indistinguishable, they become specified to form structures characteristic of particular body regions. Moreover, the characteristic development of specific vertebrae seems to be related to the intrinsic properties of their particular somatic precursor. Somites transplanted to another region will form structures typical of the region of their origin. Thoracic somites transplanted to the lumbar region, for example, form typical thoracic vertebrae and ribs at the ectopic lumbar site. Based on experiments such as these, it has been suggested that somites acquire their regional specificity during early stages of segmentation.[1]
>
> The somites first appear in the future occipital region of the embryo. They soon develop craniocaudally and give rise to most of the axial skeleton (bones of the cranium, vertebral column, ribs, and sternum) and associated musculature, as well as to the adjacent dermis of the skin. The first pair of somites appears at the end of the third week a short distance caudal to the cranial end of the notochord. Subsequent pairs form in a craniocaudal sequence.[2]

If one remembers that the structures derived from the axial core include the cranium, vertebral column, paravertebral muscles, ribs and sternum, it becomes more apparent why a lateral strain pattern at the sphenobasilar junction in the cranium results in scoliosis. To correct the scoliosis, this lateral strain pattern must be addressed first in order to facilitate treatment of the spine, ribcage, and sternum. In our experience, one of the least common causes of congenital scoliosis, though it is frequently blamed for this problem, is a hemivertebra.

> The developing vertebral bodies have two chondrification centers that soon unite. A hemivertebra results from failure of one of the chondrification centers to appear and subsequent failure of half of the vertebra to form. These defective vertebrae produce scoliosis (lateral curvature) of the vertebral column.[3]

Because ossification of typical vertebrae begins during the embryonic period and usually ends by the twenty-fifth year, there is a very large window of opportunity for treating abnormal curvatures of the spine and deformities of the head.

In order to successfully treat the spine, there are a few basic anatomical features that need to be considered. The atlanto-occipital joint consists of two condyles on the occiput that glide in the two concavities on the atlas, allowing for nodding of the head. The atlas rotates around the odontoid process like a wheel on its axle, allowing rotation of the head. In the remainder of the spine, the facets overlap like shingles on a roof. The simplicity of the embryonic development of the back and neck works greatly to the physician's advantage when treating the spine because these three different types of anatomical joints respond to the same treatment vector force, that is, an anterior and superior force along the functional planes of the sclerotomes. The degree of angle of this treatment vector is strictly dictated by the region of the spine being treated—lumbar, thoracic, or cervical.

## A Simple Way to Diagnose Spinal Dysfunctions

With the patient standing, run the pads of your thumbs (using some pressure) down the spine approximately one inch on either side of the spinous processes and feel for the following:

1. A bump on each side, indicating that both facets are in flexion or forward-bending (flexion dysfunction)

2. A dent on each side, indicating that both facets are in extension or backward-bending (extension dysfunction)

3. A bump on one side and dent on the other, indicating that the facet joint on one side is in flexion and the other is in extension (side-bending and rotation dysfunction)

4. Tension, muscle spasm, and lack of mobility, but no bump or dent at the facet joints, indicating vertical compression of the facets of the vertebrae (compression dysfunction)

*Note*: All areas of the spine are treated in a similar manner, that is, the vector force is usually generated anteriorly and superiorly toward the patient's eyes. Balanced tension is maintained along this vector until the release occurs.

This is true regardless of the type of dysfunction: flexion, extension, side-bending and rotation, or compression. The angle and magnitude of the anterior and superior vector force varies only with the type of vertebrae being treated (cervical, thoracic, or lumbar).

For treating severe areas of somatic dysfunction of the spine that require maintaining an anterior and superior vector force that exceeds the endurance of your hands, the BackMaster® thoracic and lumbar devices have been developed.[4] These devices will maintain the specific vector force as long as is necessary to achieve release of even the most stubborn dysfunctions. They can be used in the physician's office to save wear and tear on the hands and/or used by patients at home.

## *Whiplash Injuries*

The initial, major force in a rear-end collision is in the vertical direction. When the thoracic kyphosis and lumbar lordosis are flattened suddenly because of the impact with the car seat, the spine lengthens, driving the atlas up into the occiput and the sacrum down into the pelvis. Then the head whips backward, straining the anterior fascia and muscles. Hence, the patient has neck pain and lower back pain.

The treatment protocol for someone who has suffered from a whiplash injury is to treat the entire spine, including the sacrum, as described in this chapter. Then treat the anterior cervical fascia and the bowstring fascia, as described in Chapter 9. The falciform and coronary fascia which attach to the liver need to be treated as well. The liver is a heavy organ, which may be pulled out of its normal position due to an acceleration-and-deceleration injury.

## *Lumbar and Lower Thoracic Spine*

TECHNIQUE: Supine indirect ligamentous articular release

SYMPTOMS/DIAGNOSIS: Lower back pain and/or radicular pain down a lower extremity

PATIENT: Supine

PHYSICIAN: Seated at the side of the table just below the level of the sacrum and facing the patient's head. *Note:* If you are right-handed, sit on the patient's right, and if you are left-handed, on the patient's left.

PROCEDURE: Grasp the patient's sacrum with your dominant hand. Grasp the vertebra to be treated with your other hand transverse to the longitudinal axis of the spine. The finger pads of your nondominant hand are just lateral to the far paravertebral muscles, and your thenar eminence is at the lateral edge of the near paravertebral muscles. First, bring the sacrum to a balance point. This may involve moving it superiorly or inferiorly while side-bending and/or rotating as necessary. Then carry the affected vertebra anteriorly and superiorly toward the patient's eyes, which is almost always the position of ease. ("Position of ease" refers to the direction the fascia moves most easily.) Maintain the sacrum and the affected vertebra at their balance points until a release occurs in both areas. This technique treats the sacrum at the same time the lumbar spine is being treated. If there are several areas of dysfunction, start at the lowest area and work up toward the head. If there is only lumbar or lower thoracic dysfunction, that is, the sacrum is not affected, you can use just the hand on the lumbar or thoracic vertebra to treat that segment.

**Figure 7.1** Lumbar and lower thoracic spine hand positions

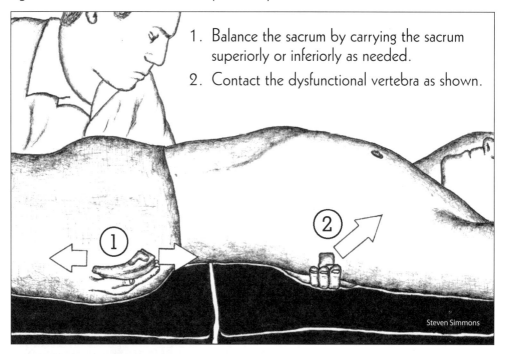

1. Balance the sacrum by carrying the sacrum superiorly or inferiorly as needed.
2. Contact the dysfunctional vertebra as shown.

Steven Simmons

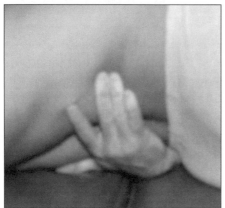

**Figure 7.2** The patient has been rolled to the side so that you can see the hand placement across the paravertebrals. Note that there should be a hand on the sacrum. The treatment is with the patient supine.

**Figure 7.3**  The patient has been rolled to the side so that you can see the hand placement across the paravertebrals. The treatment is with the patient supine.

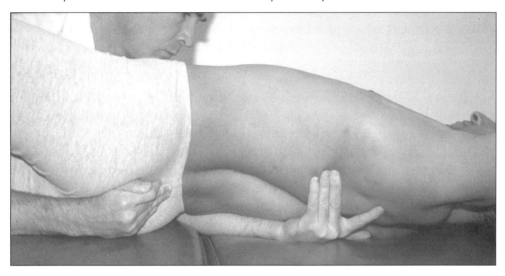

**Figure 7.4**  Lumbar and lower thoracic spine treatment position

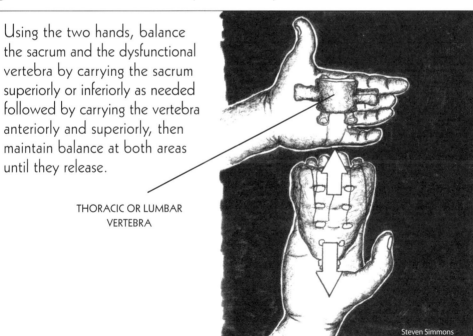

Using the two hands, balance the sacrum and the dysfunctional vertebra by carrying the sacrum superiorly or inferiorly as needed followed by carrying the vertebra anteriorly and superiorly, then maintain balance at both areas until they release.

THORACIC OR LUMBAR VERTEBRA

Steven Simmons

## *Upper Thoracic Spine*

TECHNIQUE: Supine indirect ligamentous articular release

SYMPTOMS/DIAGNOSIS: Upper back pain

PATIENT: Supine

PHYSICIAN: Seated at the head of the table, facing the top of the patient's head

PROCEDURE: Slide your hands, palms up, under the patient's back from the sides. Feel for areas of dysfunction in the thoracic spine. Place the pads of your fingers approximately one-and-one-half inches on either side of the spinous process of the dysfunctional vertebra. Carry your fingertips anteriorly and superiorly, maintaining this balanced steady pressure until you feel a release occur. In this case, the firm dysfunctional area softens and the vertebra returns to its normal functioning position. If there are several areas of dysfunction, start at the lowest area and work up toward the head.

## *Cervical Spine*

TECHNIQUE: Supine indirect ligamentous articular release

SYMPTOMS/DIAGNOSIS: Neck pain, headache, loss of range of motion of the neck, and radicular pain and/or numbness of the arms

PATIENT: Supine, approximately eight inches down from the edge of the table

PHYSICIAN: Sitting at the head of the table

PROCEDURE: Place the thenar eminences of your supine hands under both sides of the back of the head along the surface projection of the tentorium cerebelli.With the pads of your middle fingers approximately one-half inch apart, reach down the neck as far as you can and contact the lowest cervical dysfunction you can reach. If your fingers are long enough, you can even treat the upper thoracic vertebrae. Draw your finger pads anteriorly and superiorly below the area of dysfunction, slightly flexing your hands to draw your fingers toward the thenar eminences while maintaining contact with the head. Maintain the balanced compression between your contact points across the tentorium cerebelli and the area of dysfunction in the spine until a release occurs. If there is more than one area of dysfunction, slide your finger pads superiorly until they contact the next area of dysfunction, then repeat this process.

The following should be noted:

1. The atlanto-axial joint is treated exactly as described above for the cervical spine.

2. The atlanto-occipital joint is treated exactly as described above for the cervical spine except that the fingertips are used on the atlas, instead of the finger pads. The fingertips are carried anteriorly and superiorly toward the patient's eyes until the atlas glides forward on the occipital condyles.

3. Once the atlanto-occipital joint has been released by bringing it to a still point and then allowing it to make a change, you have completed a compression of the fourth ventricle of the brain.[5] This freeing of the tentorium cerebelli releases the occiput, parietal bone, and temporal bone, allowing them to move in synchrony with the cranial rhythmic impulse.

**Figure 7.5** Cervical spine hand position

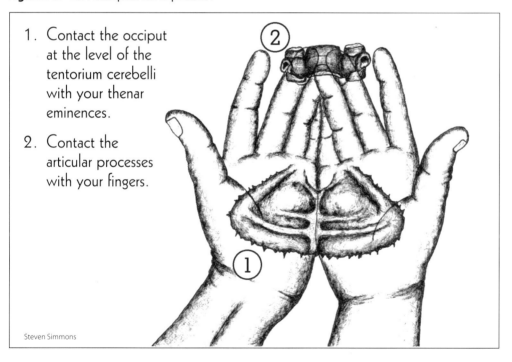

1. Contact the occiput at the level of the tentorium cerebelli with your thenar eminences.

2. Contact the articular processes with your fingers.

Steven Simmons

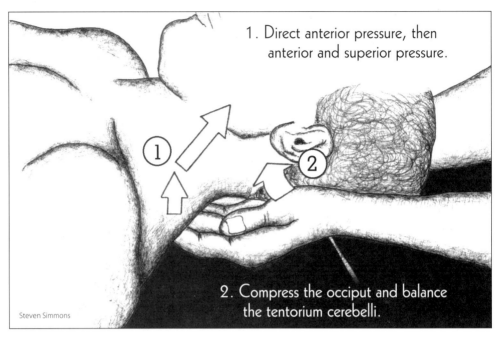

1. Direct anterior pressure, then anterior and superior pressure.

2. Compress the occiput and balance the tentorium cerebelli.

Steven Simmons

**Figure 7.6** Cervical spine technique

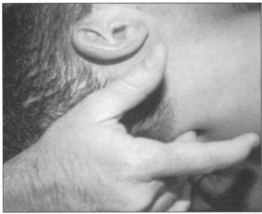

**Figure 7.7** Cervical spine treatment hand position. Note that the patient's head is turned so you can see the hand placement. The head is supine during the treatment.

1   Larsen, William, J., Human Embryology, 2nd ed., New York: Churchill Livingston Inc., 1997, p. 97.

2   Moore, Keith L., and Persaud, T. V. N., The Developing Human, Clinically Oriented Embryology, 6th ed., Philadelphia: W. B. Saunders Co., 1998, p. 74.

3   Ibid, p. 418.

4   The BackMaster® Thoracic and Lumbar Devices are available from Back-Jack, Inc., 10622 Garland Rd., Dallas, Texas 75218. Phone: (214) 324-8877.

5   Magoun, Harold I., Osteopathy in the Cranial Field, 3rd ed., Indianapolis, IN: The Cranial Academy, 1976.

CHAPTER EIGHT

# Upper Extremities

## *Anterior Cervical Fascia and Anterior Scalene Muscles*

The anterior cervical fascia is attached to the base of the skull, hyoid bone, scapula, clavicle, and sternum. Through the pretracheal fascia, the anterior cervical fascia is connected to the fibrous pericardium and then to the diaphragm. The anterior cervical fascia surrounds the pharynx, larynx, and thyroid gland. It forms the carotid sheath, and via the prevertebral fascia, the anterior cervical fascia is connected to the tissue that surrounds the trachea and esophagus. Therefore, the anterior cervical fascia is concerned directly with lymphatic drainage of the head, neck, thorax, and upper extremities. Strains in the anterior cervical fascia can also affect the nerve supply to the upper extremities by impinging on the brachial plexus.

Holding a heavy object directly in front commonly causes a strained anterior cervical fascia. Examples include holding a heavy book in front of you while reading or carrying a heavy box.

TECHNIQUE: Supine direct myofascial release

SYMPTOMS/DIAGNOSIS: Globus hystericus, headache, pain or numbness in the arm or hand on the affected side, pain medial to shoulder blade on the affected side, or tightness in the supraclavicular fossa

PATIENT: Supine

PHYSICIAN: Seated at the head of the table, facing the patient's feet

PROCEDURE: Place the pads of your thumbs in the supraclavicular fossa on either side of the sternal notch, just lateral to the sternocleidomastoid muscles. Press your thumbs inferiorly, straight toward the patient's feet. Treat the tight side with balanced pressure. Your other thumb may be removed. (Both sides may be tight; in that case, both sides can be treated at the same time.) Once the tightness in the tissue under your thumbs dissipates, draw the pads of your thumbs laterally toward the acromioclavicular joints. The tight fascia and anterior scalene muscles will "melt" ahead of your thumbs. This area is very sensitive, so take great care to use the exact amount of balanced pressure necessary to achieve the release. If you let the patient know that you are aware of this tenderness, he or she can better tolerate the discomfort until the release occurs.

It should be noted that:

1. Releasing the anterior cervical fascia will result in a release of the anterior scalene and the omohyoid muscles.

2. Always press directly with the pads of your thumbs. In this case, the pads of your thumbs are parallel to the clavicles and pointed toward the sternoclavicular joint. Avoid pushing your thumbs sideways, as this would sprain the distal joints of your thumbs.

**Figure 8.1** Anterior cervical fascia technique

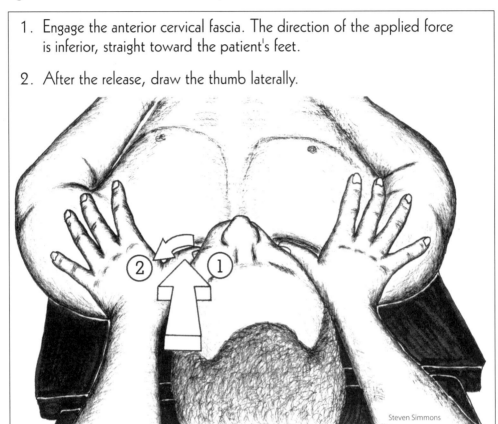

1. Engage the anterior cervical fascia. The direction of the applied force is inferior, straight toward the patient's feet.

2. After the release, draw the thumb laterally.

Steven Simmons

## *Middle and Posterior Scalene Muscles and Levator Scapulae*

TECHNIQUE: Supine direct myofascial release

SYMPTOMS/DIAGNOSIS: Pain in lateral or posterior neck, headache, and pain and/or numbness in the hands or arms

PATIENT: Supine

PHYSICIAN: Seated at the head of the table, facing the patient's feet and slightly angled toward the affected side of the patient's neck

PROCEDURE: To release tight middle and posterior scalene muscles, move the pad of your thumb directly posterior to the anterior scalene muscle you just treated in the pervious technique. Locate the tight middle or posterior scalene muscle and apply steady medial and inferior pressure to the affected muscle until the spasm releases. Moving even further posteriorly, just above the point of the scapula, the levator scapulae muscle can be released with steady medial, inferior, and slightly anterior pressure. Maintain steady pressure until the spasm releases.

**Figure 8.2**  Scalenes technique

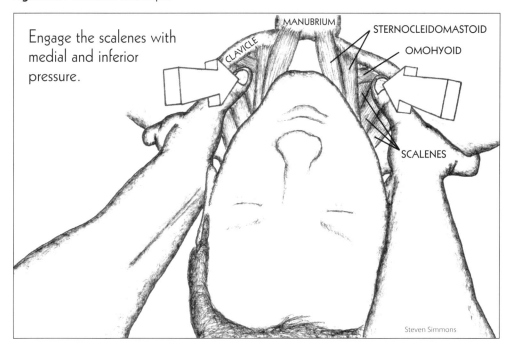

**Figure 8.3**  Scalenes hand position

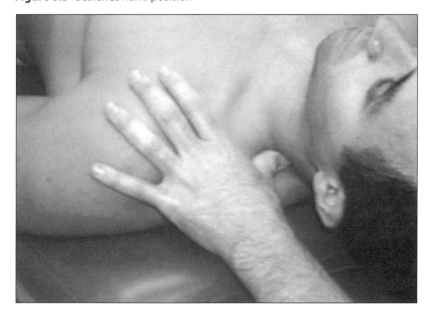

## *Clavicle*

TECHNIQUE: Seated direct ligamentous articular release

SYMPTOMS/DIAGNOSIS: Pain at either end of the clavicle

PATIENT: Seated on the side of the table

PHYSICIAN: Seated on a stool slightly lower than the patient, facing the patient

PROCEDURE: Place the tip of one thumb on the medial and inferior portion of the medial end of the clavicle. Place your other thumb just medial and inferior to the distal end of the clavicle. Have the patient drape the forearm of the affected side across your upper arm on that side. Carry both your thumbs laterally, superiorly, and slightly posteriorly while the patient draws the unaffected shoulder posteriorly. Maintain a balanced lateral, superior, and posterior pressure with both thumbs until a release is felt and the clavicle moves laterally and posteriorly.

**Figure 8.4** Clavicle technique

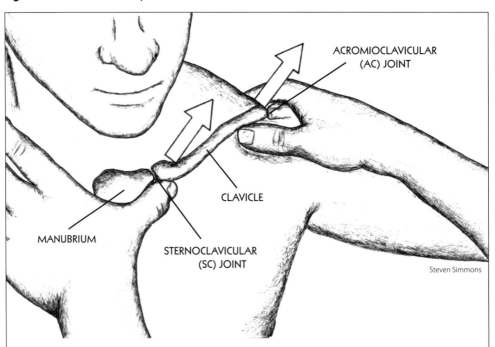

MANUBRIUM

CLAVICLE

STERNOCLAVICULAR (SC) JOINT

ACROMIOCLAVICULAR (AC) JOINT

Steven Simmons

Contact the clavicle just lateral to the sternoclavicular joint with one thumb and just medial to the acromioclavicular joint with the other thumb. Carry both your thumbs laterally, superiorly, and slightly posteriorly. Maintain a balanced tension with both thumbs until a release is felt.

# Shoulders

## A Common Mechanism of Shoulder Injury

One of the most common mechanisms of shoulder injury is initiated by a spasm in the teres minor muscle that draws the humerus to the posterior inferior portion of the glenoid fossa. This leaves a gap at the anterior and superior glenohumeral joint, allowing the humerus to pinch the subdeltoid bursa when the arm is raised.

The most common mechanism that causes a spasm in the teres minor muscle is reaching posteriorly. Examples include reaching back into the rear seat for an item while seated in the front seat of the car, reaching back to put on a coat or hook a bra, or slipping on ice and reaching back to catch oneself.

## Shoulder Treatment Sequence

The key to treating shoulder dysfunctions (subdeltoid bursitis, frozen shoulder, and/or pain at the point of the shoulder) is to first release the spasm in the teres minor muscle followed by recentering the humerus in the glenoid fossa.

### *Teres Minor*

TECHNIQUE: Lateral recumbent direct myofascial release

SYMPTOMS/DIAGNOSIS: Pain at the anterior superior aspect of the shoulder, pain in the posterior axillary fold, or restricted shoulder range of motion

PATIENT: Lateral recumbent position with the affected shoulder up

PHYSICIAN: Standing at the side of the table, behind the patient

PROCEDURE: Locate the teres minor muscle at the posterior axillary fold. With the pad of your thumb at right angles to the fibers of the muscle, press at the point of maximum spasm, maintaining steady pressure superiorly, medially, and slightly anteriorly until you feel the spasm release.

**Figure 8.5** Teres minor technique

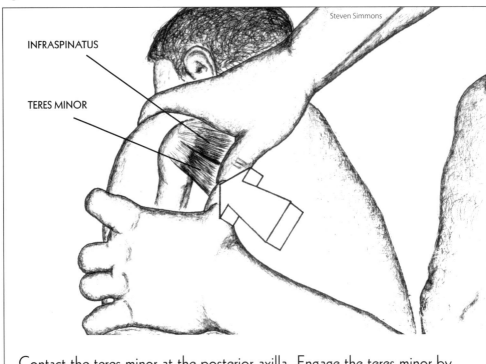

Steven Simmons

INFRASPINATUS

TERES MINOR

Contact the teres minor at the posterior axilla. Engage the teres minor by directing pressure superiorly, medially, and slightly anteriorly. Maintain balanced pressure until a release is felt.

## *Recentering the Head of the Humerus in the Glenoid Fossa*

TECHNIQUE: Lateral recumbent direct ligamentous articular release

SYMPTOMS/DIAGNOSIS: Pain at the anterior superior aspect of the shoulder, pain in the posterior axillary fold, or restricted shoulder range of motion

PATIENT: Lateral recumbent position with the affected shoulder up

PHYSICIAN: Standing at the side of the table, behind the patient

PROCEDURE: Once the teres minor muscle has been released, cup the elbow in the palm of your hand with the patient's arm bent and relaxed. With your other hand (the one closest to the patient's head), grasp the shoulder at the glenohumeral joint. Controlling the humerus from the elbow, draw the elbow laterally and slightly anteriorly or posteriorly to bring balanced tension through the shoulder. Then hold steady compression on the humerus into the glenoid fossa while you oppose this pressure with your hand on the shoulder. While compressing your hands toward each other, you may need to adjust the direction of your forces on the glenoid fossa anteriorly or posteriorly in order to feel the maximum rigidity between your two hands. The resulting force will resemble the shape of a hockey stick, with the elbow being the top end and the opposite shoulder on the table being the tip of the blade. When the release occurs, the head of the humerus will move superiorly and anteriorly in the glenoid fossa. The shaft of the humerus will move superiorly and sweep anteriorly past the patient's ear.

In the above treatment, you are balancing the force exerted through the tip of the elbow with the force going through the glenoid fossa. This brings your two hands toward each other and directs the force from the elbow into the table through the other shoulder. If the elbow at the balance point is slightly anterior to the patient's body, the hand on the shoulder will be compressing the shoulder slightly anteriorly while you are compressing superiorly and slightly posteriorly on the elbow. Conversely, if the elbow at the balance point is slightly posterior to the patient, the hand on the shoulder will be drawing traction toward the physician. The pressure through the shaft of the humerus is fairly firm.

**Figure 8.6** Humerus technique

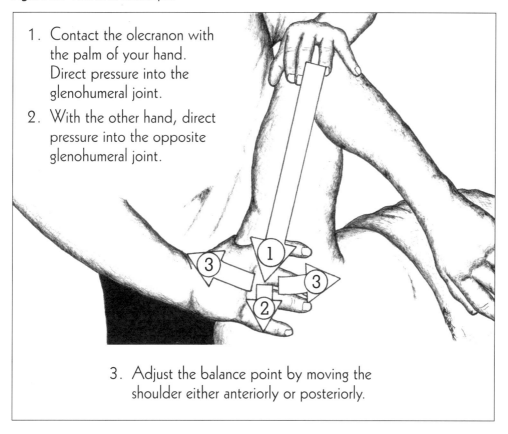

1. Contact the olecranon with the palm of your hand. Direct pressure into the glenohumeral joint.

2. With the other hand, direct pressure into the opposite glenohumeral joint.

3. Adjust the balance point by moving the shoulder either anteriorly or posteriorly.

# Anterior Shoulder

## *Pectoralis Major Muscle*

TECHNIQUE: Supine direct myofascial release

SYMPTOMS/DIAGNOSIS: Pain in the front of the shoulder, or shoulder drawn anteriorly

PATIENT: Supine

PHYSICIAN: Seated at the side of the table, level with the patient's waist, and facing head of table

PROCEDURE: On the side of the spasm, grasp the patient's hand with your hand that is farthest from the patient's body. Draw the arm approximately 30° lateral to the patient's side. Using the pad of the thumb of your medial hand, contact the pectoralis major muscle in the anterior axillary fold approximately two inches from its insertion on the humerus. Usually this is the point of maximum spasm. Apply balanced pressure with the pad of your thumb at right angles to the muscle's fibers just medial to the tendon while drawing slight traction on the patient's arm with your other hand. Maintain steady, balanced pressure until you feel a release of the spasm.

## *Pectoralis Minor Muscle, Coracobrachialis Muscle, and the Short Head of the Biceps Brachii*

TECHNIQUE: Supine direct myofascial release

SYMPTOMS/DIAGNOSIS: Pain in the front of the shoulder, or the shoulder drawn anteriorly

PATIENT: Supine

PHYSICIAN: Standing at the side of the table at midchest level, facing the head of the table

PROCEDURE: If a spasm is noted in the pectoralis minor muscle, maintain steady, balanced pressure medially with the tip of the pad of the thumb of your dominant hand, starting at the lateral edge of the pectoralis minor muscle approximately two inches below the coracoid process. Maintain steady pressure across the fibers sweeping medially across the upper chest wall as the muscle relaxes ahead of your thumb.

Treat the coracobrachialis muscle and the short head of the biceps brachii with a similar technique. Move your thumbs just lateral and inferior to the coracoid process and apply a steady, balanced pressure in a medial and posterior direction.

## *Subclavius Muscles, Costocoracoid Ligaments, Costoclavicular Ligaments, and Upper Mediastinum*

TECHNIQUE: Supine direct ligamentous articular release

SYMPTOMS/DIAGNOSIS: Pain in front of the shoulder, or the shoulder drawn anteriorly

PATIENT: Supine

PHYSICIAN: Standing at the side of the table at midchest level, facing the head of the table

PROCEDURE: If you note a spasm in the subclavius muscles and/or strain in the costocoracoid and costoclavicular ligaments, compress toward the table while grasping across the subclavicular spaces with the pad of your thumb in the near fossa and the pad of your middle finger in the far fossa. Press posteriorly and contract your hand, drawing your thumb and middle finger together. Maintain this balanced contraction until you feel a release of the tensions in both fossae and your thumb and middle finger move toward each other.

**Figure 8.7** Anterior shoulder anatomy

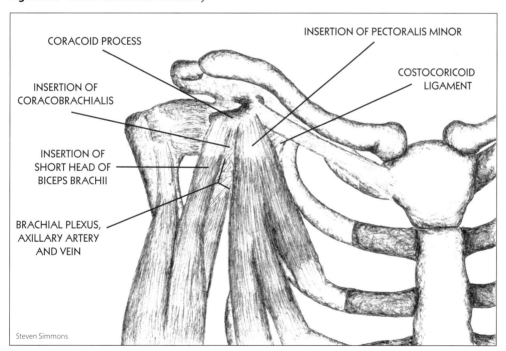

CORACOID PROCESS

INSERTION OF PECTORALIS MINOR

COSTOCORICOID LIGAMENT

INSERTION OF CORACOBRACHIALIS

INSERTION OF SHORT HEAD OF BICEPS BRACHII

BRACHIAL PLEXUS, AXILLARY ARTERY AND VEIN

Steven Simmons

**Figure 8.8** Coracobrachialis muscle and short head of biceps brachii (anterior shoulder) technique

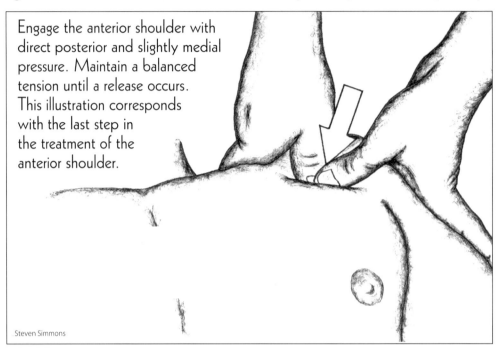

Engage the anterior shoulder with direct posterior and slightly medial pressure. Maintain a balanced tension until a release occurs. This illustration corresponds with the last step in the treatment of the anterior shoulder.

Steven Simmons

**Figure 8.9** Anterior shoulder hand position

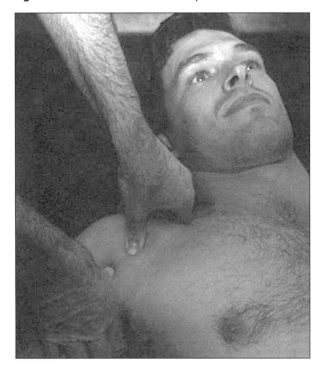

# Tennis Elbow and Related Injuries

Strains in the interosseous membrane between the radius and ulna affect the elbow. Thus, if there is a strain in the interosseous membrane, both the wrist and elbow are usually involved. To get the forearm working properly, both ends should be treated.

## *Forearm and Elbow*

TECHNIQUE: Supine, seated, or standing direct ligamentous articular release

SYMPTOMS/DIAGNOSIS: Elbow pain or stiffness (loss of motion)

PATIENT: Supine, seated, or standing

PHYSICIAN: Standing slightly in front and on the side of the affected elbow, facing the patient

PROCEDURE: Start with the patient's elbow bent to 90°. Grasp the patient's olecranon process with your thumb and index finger. Both the thumb and index finger should be at the proximal tip of the olecranon process, with your thumb and fingertip just on the edge of the grooves on either side of the olecranon process, and the index finger on the medial aspect of the olecranon process. With your other hand, grasp the dorsum of the patient's fully-flexed wrist. Rotate the patient's forearm into full pronation.

Compress the forearm between your two hands, drawing the patient's elbow toward complete extension. If a dysfunction is present, you will notice a firm barrier against bringing the arm into full extension. Maintain steady, balanced pressure against this barrier until the elbow straightens and your thumb and fingertip slide through the grooves on either side of the olecranon process. At this point, the treatment is complete. It has resolved torsional strains of the radial head, and lateral or medial deviation of the olecranon process in the olecranon groove (that is, lateral or medial deviation of the ulna on the humerus).

**Figure 8.10** Forearm technique

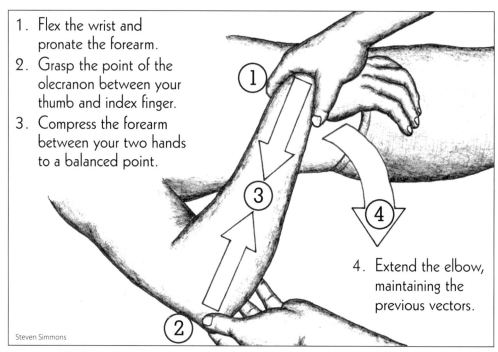

1. Flex the wrist and pronate the forearm.
2. Grasp the point of the olecranon between your thumb and index finger.
3. Compress the forearm between your two hands to a balanced point.
4. Extend the elbow, maintaining the previous vectors.

Steven Simmons

## *Carpal Tunnel*

Normally, the hand deviates in the ulnar direction from the forearm by approximately 15° to 30°. Strains of the interosseous membrane of the forearm result in a loss of this normal carrying angle, or, in extreme cases, the hand is maintained in radial deviation. The result is compression of the carpal tunnel between the distal heads of the radius and ulna. To treat carpal tunnel syndrome, you must resolve the strain of the interosseous membrane between the radius and ulna as well as the ligaments of the wrist. By releasing strains in the fascia of the forearm and wrist, pressure on the ulnar nerve can also be relieved. This technique addresses both the interosseous membrane and the ligaments of the wrist at the same time.

It is important to note that:

1. When the dysfunction in the wrist and forearm has been corrected, the patient must be instructed on how to ergonomically use his or her hand to avoid reinjuring it. The hand must be maintained in 15° to 30° ulnar deviation when performing any task to avoid a repeat of carpal tunnel syndrome.

2. When treating the wrist, it is important to also treat the elbow as described above.

3. Since carpal tunnel affects more than just the wrist, the upper thoracic region must be treated as well.

TECHNIQUE: Supine, seated, or standing combined ligamentous articular release

SYMPTOMS/DIAGNOSIS: Numbness and/or pain in the wrist, hand, or fingers (usually the thumb, index finger, middle finger, and lateral half of the ring finger)

PATIENT: Supine, seated, or standing

PHYSICIAN: Seated or standing on the affected side, facing the patient

PROCEDURE: Assume that the patient has carpal tunnel in the right arm. (Reverse the technique for the left arm.) With the patient's right hand in full supination, grasp the hypothenar side with your left hand, your fingertips in the patient's palm. Reach across with your right hand (as if you are going to shake hands) and grasp the patient's thumb, wrapping your fingers around it. Push the wrist into full flexion with your grip on the thumb. Draw the hand into full radial deviation with your grip on the hypothenar side of the patient's hand. Now, with both hands maintaining full flexion and full radial deviation, start rotating the patient's hand from supination toward pronation (palm down). When you meet a barrier in the pronation process, maintain steady pressure against that barrier until it dissipates. When you feel the barrier melt, allow the hand to come out of flexion, bringing it around into full pronation and ulnar deviation (toward the little finger).

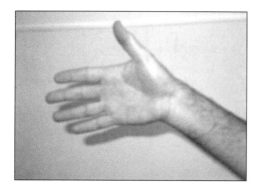

**Figure 8.11** Normal angle of the wrist

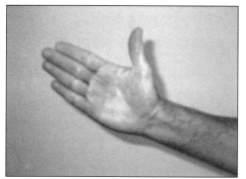

**Figure 8.12** Abnormal angle of the wrist, which is how patients will present with carpal tunnel

**Figure 8.13** Carpal tunnel technique, first diagram

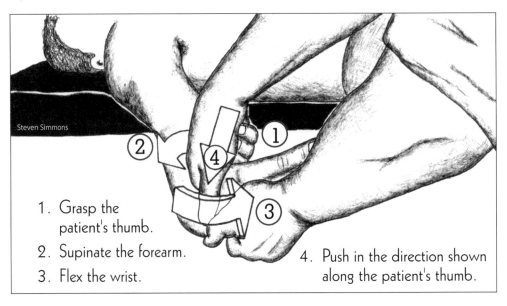

Steven Simmons

1. Grasp the patient's thumb.
2. Supinate the forearm.
3. Flex the wrist.
4. Push in the direction shown along the patient's thumb.

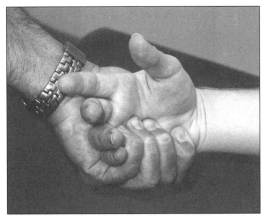

**Figure 8.14** Carpal tunnel Technique: beginning hand position

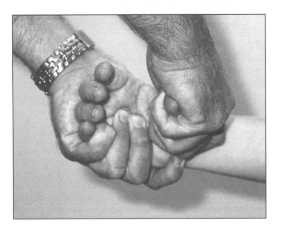

**Figure 8.15** Carpal tunnel technique. Notice that you grab the thumb with one hand while taking the hypothenar eminence with the other hand.

**Figure 8.16** Carpal tunnel technique, second diagram

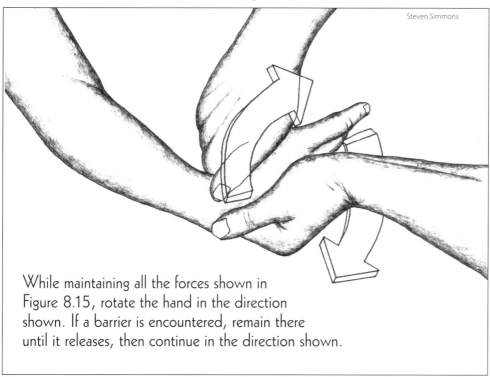

Steven Simmons

While maintaining all the forces shown in
Figure 8.15, rotate the hand in the direction
shown. If a barrier is encountered, remain there
until it releases, then continue in the direction shown.

**Figure 8.17** Carpal tunnel technique, third diagram

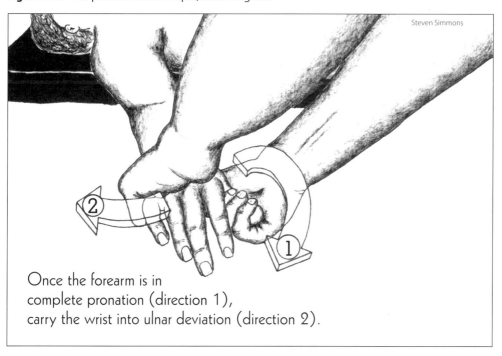

Steven Simmons

Once the forearm is in
complete pronation (direction 1),
carry the wrist into ulnar deviation (direction 2).

## *Phalanges*

*Note:* This technique also works well for treating the toes.

TECHNIQUE: Supine combined ligamentous articular release

SYMPTOMS/DIAGNOSIS: Pain and/or restricted motion in the fingers

PATIENT: Supine

PHYSICIAN: Seated or standing

PROCEDURE: Stabilize the patient's hand in pronation with your nondominant hand. Grasp the finger to be treated just distal to the proximal interphalangeal joint, with your thumb on the dorsum and your index finger on the palmar surface of the middle phalanx. Dorsiflex the proximal phalanx at the knuckle while palmar flexing the middle phalanx at the proximal interphalangeal joint. While compressing the proximal phalanx into the knuckle, medially and laterally deviate the proximal phalanx. With the proximal phalanx deviated in the direction of ease, carry the proximal phalanx laterally or medially to the barrier obstructing its movement in that direction. Maintain steady, balanced pressure against that barrier until it releases, allowing the phalanx to move equally in both directions at the knuckle.

**Figure 8.18** Phalanges technique

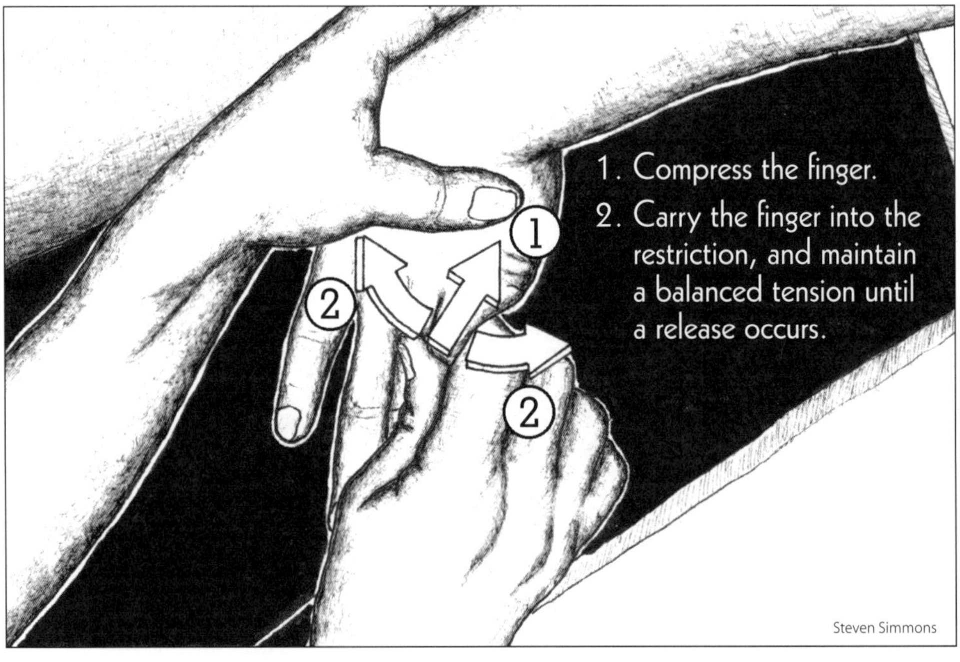

1. Compress the finger.
2. Carry the finger into the restriction, and maintain a balanced tension until a release occurs.

Steven Simmons

# SECTION III

# Integration

Human beings are more than the sum of our parts. As A.T. Still first put it, the human is a triad with mind, body, and spirit functioning together. You must learn to treat the individual parts and then evaluate the work to see that everything is functioning together. If any one part is dysfunctional, it will affect one's health. Learn to treat the individual parts, and then learn the interconnections and interrelationships among those parts. The mind can be affected greatly by changes in the tissue. Release of somatic dysfunction can bring back memories and emotions. Wilhelm Reich documented this in the 1930s,[1] and John Upledger[2] discussed this phenomenon in his books on craniosacral therapy, calling it somatoemotional release. Robert Fulford also stated, in one of the last courses he taught, that when we treat the body we also treat the spirit.[3] Now that you know how to treat the individual areas of the body, shift to a global view utilizing the information presented in the following section to treat the entire body.

This section deals with the bowstring, diaphragms, and the key lesion. The bowstring connects and coordinates the movement of the diaphragms, which in turn augment the flow of the interstitial fluid. The rhythmic flow of the interstitial fluid bathes the individual cells and provides them with nutrients and removal of waste products. By definition, the key lesion is the major obstacle to the movement of the interstitial fluid. By addressing the key lesion early in the treatment session, you can expedite the treatment. By adjusting your overall treatment sequence, you can improve the efficiency of the treatment sessions.

The most reasonable and commonly asked questions concern where to start a treatment and when to end it. The approach that we teach is:

1. Find and treat the key lesion, which removes the largest barrier to the rhythmic flow of the interstitial fluid.

2. If the spine exhibits a somatic dysfunction, check the anterior fascia of the bowstring. Treat any anterior dysfunction found. Then check and see if any posterior ones remain and treat those using the previously discussed techniques.

3. Check the eight diaphragms from the feet up or the head down. Treat any dysfunction using the techniques prevously discussed.

In addition, as always, document your findings.

# CHAPTER NINE

# Key Lesion

The key lesion is the primary or most important dysfunction in the body and may well be the injury that prevented the patient's natural healing mechanism from effectively dealing with any ensuing injuries. This dysfunction acts like a beaver's dam across a stream. If the dam is removed, the water will flow downstream unimpeded. Likewise, if the key lesion can be removed, the rest of the body's dysfunctions may resolve themselves or be easily handled by the physician.

There are many different methods you can use for locating the key lesion.

When looking for motion or lack of motion, try not to focus directly on the patient; instead, keep the patient in your peripheral vision, which utilizes more rods than cones. Rods are better at detecting motion. This will assist you in locating the areas that are not moving—these are the areas of dysfunction. One of these areas will be the key lesion.

# Searching for the Key Lesion

Before we describe the four methods for finding the key lesion, it should be noted that we primarily use methods two through four, described below, to determine where we are going to start our treatment. This we do as part of our standard osteopathic exam.

## Method 1

Do a systematic search through the body, and treat all the dysfunctions you encounter until you locate and treat the key lesion. It is usually the oldest and most significant dysfunction and prevents the other dysfunctions from resolving. This is a solid but very time-consuming method. You might have to treat a patient for one or two hours before you find the key lesion.

## Method 2

Observe the patient walking toward and away from you to locate the areas that are not moving. These will be like axles: Everything else will be moving around them, but they will remain motionless. One of these dysfunctional areas will most likely be the key lesion.

When looking for these motions, whether the patient is walking or standing still, try not to focus directly on the patient for the reasons mentioned above. This will help you pick up the motion. Once you have located the key lesion, try to attack it first because it will probably take the longest to treat but will produce the most benefit. You would hate to see it emerge last!

## Method 3

Pull gently on one leg to determine if there is an area of restriction further up in the body. This is done while standing at the foot of the table. (The feeling is that of pulling on the corner of a tablecloth to determine where a nail has been driven through it, anchoring it to the table.) Now, pull on the other leg and see if it gives you the same information. The most restricted area will most likely be the key lesion. This method is also discussed in other texts.[4]

### *Method 4*

Observe the patient getting up from a chair and getting onto the treatment table. This may reveal additional restrictions of motion that you could not find while watching the patient walk. For example, watching a patient push on his thighs when rising from a chair will indicate a psoas muscle spasm. If the patient bends to one side, the psoas muscle spasm is located only on that side, but if the patient bends straight forward, the problem is bilateral.

# Summary

The parts that do not move are relatively hard, while those that do move are soft. You do not have to toss the parts around and do a lot of range of motion tests. Feel the body. The parts that are hard are the problem, and the soft parts are normal. Likewise, any part of the body that does not move has a problem.

The purpose of the treatments discussed in this book is to soften what is hard. It does not really matter how you accomplish this. What is important is that you do the techniques until the area softens and starts to move. This is a change that happens very quickly, in a split second. If you stop one second before the change occurs, you have done nothing, absolutely nothing! You have not affected the tissues in the slightest. For example, while it is unusual, it may take ten minutes for a change to occur. In this case, if you only held the tension for nine minutes and fifty-nine seconds, nothing would happen and the patient would gain no benefit. If you had held it for one more second, the change would have occurred. Of course, most treatments do not take ten minutes, but the point is that if you stop before the change has occurred, you have accomplished nothing.

In the next two chapters we will discuss the bowstring and treatment of the diaphragms. The bowstring is a systematic treatment method for the anterior fascia of the body. It is used and checked when there is pain in the anterior body and to prevent spinal dysfunction from spontaneously returning.

When do we check all the diaphragms? After we have treated the key lesions, because we want to make sure that the cranial rhythmic impulse is moving through the whole body.

The term key lesion is used because, when it is corrected, it is like using a key to unlock the rest of the body's dysfunctions.

The normal healthy human body is supple and flexible, with the interstitial fluid flowing freely to and fro in all areas. A healthy person feels good. We do not see healthy people for OMT because they can clear all of their minor injuries on their own. If they sustain a serious injury that their body cannot resolve, we will see them eventually. If they come in early, this key lesion will be their only dysfunction. If they do not get this dysfunction resolved for years, their body will be unable to resolve any ensuing injuries. These injuries or dysfunctions stack up, causing more and more areas of rigidity and lack of mobility and lack of inherent motility. The original severe dysfunction that stopped the body from clearing the ensuing injuries is what we term the key lesion. If the patient continually returns with the same complaint, one of two things is happening. You have not resolved their key lesion or they are continuing to reinjure themselves (sitting in a recliner or couch, bending and twisting at the same time, clenching their teeth, etc.) Rollin Becker and Robert Fulford did not feel they had time to waste, so they went directly to the key lesion first. A lot of times that was all they treated. Their results speak for themselves. As Rollin Becker would put it, "Fix the engine first, then the rest of the treatment time is just chrome polishing."

If you address the key lesion first, many of the lesser lesions (dysfunctions) will be resolved by the body's own homeostatic mechanisms. The remainder will be easier for you to work with and release.

The key lesion is what prevents the patient's body from clearing dysfunctions on its own. Resolving the key lesion is essential for the patient to reach normal health. Every patient has a key lesion or they would not be in your office. Look for it early and resolve it as soon as you can. The dramatic results you will get by removing the key lesion early will astound you.

---

[1]  Reich, Wilhelm, *Character Analysis: Principles and Technique for Psychoanalyst in Practice and in Training*, Wolfe, Theodore P. (trans.), New York: Orgone Institute Press, 1945, pp. 309B321.

[2]  Upledger, John, and Vredevoogd, Jon D., *Craniosacral Therapy*, Seattle: Eastland Press, 1983, pp. 250B254.

[3]  November 1996 Introductory Percussion Hammer Course, Indianapolis, Indiana.

[4]  Upledger, John, and Vredevoogd, Jon D., op. cit., pp. 247

# CHAPTER TEN

# Bowstring

In study group sessions, Roland Becker would frequently admonish us by saying that "You cannot just treat 'backs,' you must also treat 'fronts' or the treatment of the backs won't last."

Our bodies are three dimensional, so you must think that way.

We must use what he called the "bowstring" in our treatments.

The bowstring relates to the anterior, longitudinal, interconnected fasciae that help maintain the anterior–posterior balance of the body. The bowstring, in addition, connects the eight diaphragms, discussed in Chapter 11, and coordinates their motion in the same fashion as the dura connects and coordinates the motion of the bones of the cranium and the sacrum. In fact, the bowstring actually connects to the dura in the area of the foramen magnum and continues inferiorly all the way down to the plantar fascia of the foot. Because of these and other interrelationships discussed below, dysfunctions of the bowstring must be addressed when treating the back or indeed any part of the body.

This approach of treating the whole body, and especially the bowstring, is not a new phenomenon, as can be seen in the following passage from Dr. Sutherland:

> Dr. Still regarded the body as a complex unit composed of interrelated parts working in harmony, each endowed with the inherent desire, intelligence and ability to perform its function according to the plan of a Master Mechanic. When circumstances prevent any part of the body, whether bony or soft tissue, from doing so, the effects are far reaching. Perfect health ensues when each part is in perfect adjustment and free to do its work. Dr. Still had the greatest respect for the humours and the fasciae, the nerves, vessels, viscera and all the other elements that compose the body. He had a remarkable faculty of being able to locate maladjusted tissue, of associating cause with effect, and tracing effects back to cause.

> The fasciae envelope, separate, protect and support the various structures. Not the least important of their functions is to encourage and direct the movement of tissue fluids and to promote the flow of lymph through its channels. The various layers of fascia interconnect and present a continuity from head to foot. Dr. Still recognized 'drags' on the fasciae which are caused by hypotonicity, the weight of viscera, strains and posture. Treatment to restore the normal tension, hence function, of the fascial system is extremely effective.

**Anterior Cervical Fascia**

The anterior cervical fascia is attached to the base of the skull, the mandible, hyoid, scapula, clavicle and sternum. Through the pretracheal it is connected with the fibrous pericardium, and thence with the diaphragm. It surrounds the pharynx, larynx and thyroid gland, it forms the carotid sheath, and by way of the prevertebral fascia is connected with that which surrounds the trachea and esophagus. Therefore, the cervical fascia is concerned quite directly with lymphatic drainage of the head, neck, thorax and upper extremities. Not only voluntary movements, but respiratory activity is a factor in this vital function of the fascia, moving it forward in exhalation and backward in approximation to the spine during inhalation. Restoration of free movement of the deep cervical fascia renders unnecessary much of the soft tissue treatment of the neck and helps in overcoming intrathoracic congestions.[1]

The fascia from the skull to the plantar fascia of the foot is continuous, and it is this tissue that constitutes what is referred to as the bowstring. The bowstring connects everything down the front. Think of the spine as a "bow;" if you look at it closely, it is very similar to a recurved bow. The "string" of the bow is represented by the anterior fasciae, which attaches at the base of the skull, continues down inside the clavicles, connects to the mediastinum, and follows the falciform ligament, coronary ligament, linea alba, umbilicus, median umbilical ligament, investing fascia of the bladder, to the pelvic diaphragm. The string of the bow also includes the prevertebral fascia, which extends down the front of the bodies of the vertebra and through the respiratory diaphragm. This tissue continues inferiorly as the presacral fascia, following the anterior curve of the sacrum, attaching to the second sacral segment. As the periosteum, the fascia that formed the presacral fascia continues to the pelvic diaphragm, and then proceeds down to the knees and feet. Thus, correcting the bowstring also affects other structures and organs because of the following interconnections:

1. The mediastinum attaches to the top of the respiratory diaphragm and then follows the falciform ligament into the liver, which in turn descends to the umbilicus via the round ligament of the liver.[2]

2. The median umbilical ligament, the remnant of the urachus, runs inferiorly from the umbilicus and attaches to the top of the bladder. The median umbilical ligament is continuous with the investing fascia of the bladder, which then attaches to the pelvic diaphragm.

3. The medial umbilical ligaments originate at the umbilicus and descend along the inside of the pelvis, attaching to the presacral fascia, which in turn attaches inferiorly and posteriorly to the second sacral segment and then to the pelvic diaphragm.

4. The prevertebral fascia descends from the base of the skull, just in front of the foramen magnum, down the front of the bodies of the vertebrae to the

sacrum, forming the presacral fascia. It then continues down to the second sacral segment, and from there to the pelvic diaphragm.

As you can see, the bowstring runs from the base of the skull all the way down the front of the body, attaching to the pelvic diaphragm, and then continues down to the knees and plantar fasciae. As a result, you cannot straighten out the back by treating just the back if there is a strain in the bowstring. Strains in the bowstring resemble someone pulling on the string and thereby bending the bow. If your patient's bowstring is tight, they will walk around stooped over with their head in a forward position. You must free up restricted areas of the bowstring to get them to stand up straight. Address the bowstring as you move through the treatment session, area by area. At the conclusion of the treatment session, reassess the function of the entire bowstring as well as the diaphragms. Treat any remaining dysfunctions in these areas.

In this chapter, we will discuss accessing the bowstring at the following anatomical areas:

1. Buccinator and masseter
2. Submandibular fascia and digastric muscles
3. Anterior cervical fascia
4. Sternum
5. Coronary ligament
6. Falciform ligament
7. Superior linea alba
8. Umbilicus
9. Median umbilical ligament
10. Presacral fascia
11. Iliotibial tract
12. Fibula

**Figure 10.1** Bowstring areas

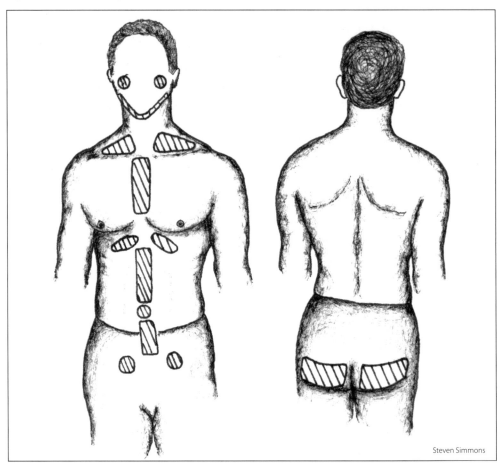

Steven Simmons

   When assessing the bowstring, one usually starts at the head and moves inferiorly to end with the plantar fascia. By starting at the head, you will not miss any major problems in the bowstring. Check each section, and if there is no dysfunction present, then move inferiorly to the next access point of the bowstring.

# Bowstring Areas

### *Buccinator and Masseter*

TECHNIQUE: Supine direct myofascial release

SYMPTOMS/DIAGNOSIS: Pain in the jaws, temporomandibular joint dysfunction, or headaches

PATIENT: Supine

PHYSICIAN: Sitting at head of table, facing the patient's feet

PROCEDURE: Contact the middle of the cheeks with the tips of your middle fingers, the pads facing the temporomandibular joints. Engage the buccinator and masseter by pressing medially until you feel the teeth, and then draw your fingertips posteriorly and slightly superiorly toward the temporo-mandibular joints. Maintain balanced tension until the buccinator and masseter muscles release bilaterally. Once the releases occur, the jaw will relax and move much more freely.

**Figure 10.2**  Buccinator and masseter technique

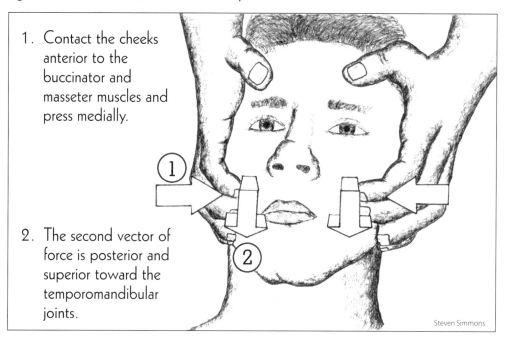

1. Contact the cheeks anterior to the buccinator and masseter muscles and press medially.

2. The second vector of force is posterior and superior toward the temporomandibular joints.

Steven Simmons

## *Submandibular Fascia and Digastric Muscles*

*Note:* This procedure also frees up the sublingual fascia.

TECHNIQUE: Supine direct myofascial release

SYMPTOMS/DIAGNOSIS: Jaw pain or spasm in the sublingual muscles

PATIENT: Supine

PHYSICIAN: Seated at head of table, facing the patient's feet

PROCEDURE: Contact the submandibular fascia and digastric muscles by curling your fingertips just beneath the chin. Using primarily the tips of your middle fingers, engage the fascia by pressing superiorly until a release is felt. Then draw your middle fingers posteriorly and laterally until they pass the angles of the jaw.

**Figure 10.3** Submandibular fascia and digastric muscles technique

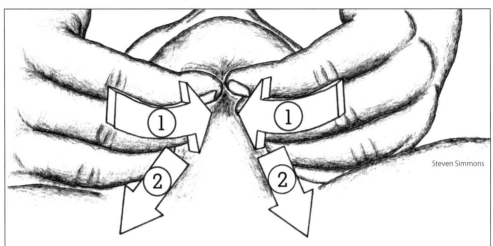

Steven Simmons

1. Engage the submandibular fascia in the direction shown.
2. Once a release is felt, move your fingertips along the medial margin as the fascia releases ahead of your fingers to just past the angle of the jaw.

## *Anterior Cervical Fascia*

TECHNIQUE: Supine direct myofascial release

SYMPTOMS/DIAGNOSIS: Globus hystericus, headache, pain or numbness in the arm or hand on the affected side, pain medial to shoulder blade on the affected side, or tightness in the supraclavicular fossa

PATIENT: Supine

PHYSICIAN: Seated at the head of the table, facing the patient's feet

PROCEDURE: Place the pads of your thumbs in the supraclavicular fossa on either side of the sternal notch, just lateral to the sternocleidomastoid muscles. Press your thumbs inferiorly, straight toward the patient's feet. Treat the tight side with balanced pressure. Your other thumb may be removed. (Both sides may be tight; in that case, both sides can be treated at the same time.) Once the tissue under your thumbs "melts," draw the pads of your thumbs laterally toward the acromioclavicular joints. The tight fascia and anterior scalene muscles will melt ahead of your thumb. This area is very sensitive, so take great care to use the exact balanced pressure necessary to achieve the release. If you let the patient know that you are aware of this tenderness, he or she can better tolerate the discomfort until the release occurs.

*Note:* Always press directly with the pads of your thumbs. In this case, the pads of your thumbs are parallel to the clavicles and point toward the sternoclavicular joint. Avoid pushing your thumbs sideways, as this would sprain the distal joint of your thumb.

**Figure 10.4**  Anterior cervical fascia technique

1. Engage the anterior cervical fascia. The direction of the applied force is inferior, straight toward the patient's feet.
2. After the release, draw the thumb laterally.

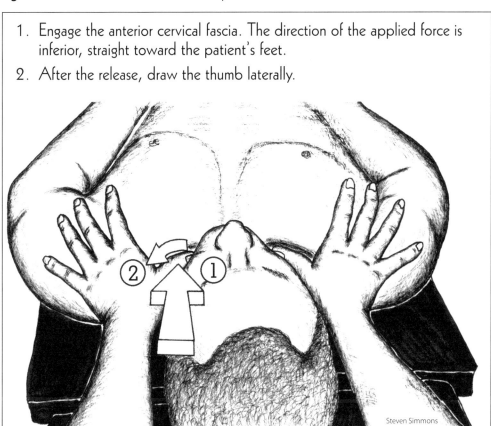

Steven Simmons

## *Sternum*

TECHNIQUE: Supine indirect ligamentous articular release

SYMPTOMS/DIAGNOSIS: Anterior midchest pain

PATIENT: Supine

PHYSICIAN: Standing at the head of the table, facing the patient's feet

PROCEDURE: Place the heel of your dominant hand on the manubrium, and grasp the body of the sternum just above the xyphoid process (the xyphosternal junction) with the pads of your fingers. Press the manubrium posteriorly and inferiorly. Contract your hand slightly to increase the flexion at the angle of Louis. If necessary, reinforce the compression with your other hand by placing it over the dorsum of the treating hand. Now that you have the sternum disengaged, see if it tips left or right. If it does tip, slightly exaggerate the tip in that direction, and maintain the tip as you try rotating the sternum clockwise and counterclockwise. Rotate in the direction of least resistance. Maintain all these vectors of force until the release occurs. The sternum should rotate back to midline, level out from side to side, and flex or extend as needed to return to its normal physiologic position. Once the release has occurred, the sternum will start flexing and extending with the "tide."

**Figure 10.5** Sternum technique

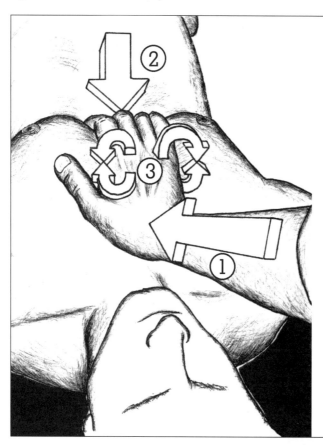

1. Contact the sternum with the heel of your hand on the manubrium and with the fingertips at the xyphosternal junction. Press in the direction shown.

2. Compress the sternum between your hand and fingertips.

3. Balance the sternum in the directions shown.

Steven Simmons

## *Coronary Ligament*

TECHNIQUE: Supine indirect myofascial release

SYMPTOMS/DIAGNOSIS: Pain in the upper left quadrant of the abdomen

PATIENT: Supine

PHYSICIAN: Standing, facing table on the right side of the patient just inferior to the diaphragm

PROCEDURE: The coronary ligament is contacted through the extraperitoneal fascia and the abdominal peritoneum just below the left costal margin, which then runs up under the respiratory diaphragm and reflects back over the liver as the coronary ligament. The contact must be made through the skin, subcutaneous fascia, and abdominal muscles until the extraperitoneal fascia and peritoneum are contacted. (Pressure can be in the 10- to 20-pound range.) The coronary ligament is treated via these tissues.[3] Place the pad of your thumb just below the left costal margin and press with balanced tension across the tight tissue you feel there in a posterior, lateral, and superior direction until a release occurs. When this happens, all the tension in this off-shoot of the coronary ligament dissipates and you will no longer be able to feel the tension. When this ligament is dysfunctional, there will often be a pulsating cardiac tug palpated, which will disappear at the release.

**Figure 10.6** Coronary ligament technique

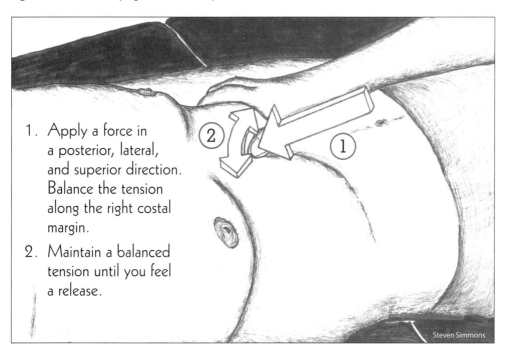

1. Apply a force in a posterior, lateral, and superior direction. Balance the tension along the right costal margin.

2. Maintain a balanced tension until you feel a release.

Steven Simmons

## *Falciform Ligament*

TECHNIQUE: Supine direct myofascial release

SYMPTOMS/DIAGNOSIS: Pain in upper right quadrant of the abdomen

PATIENT: Supine

PHYSICIAN: Standing, facing the table on the patient's left just inferior to the diaphragm

PROCEDURE: To locate the falciform ligament, place the pad of your thumb parallel to the right lower costal margin, approximately one-half to one inch below the xyphoid process, and just to the right of the midline. Press with balanced tension across the falciform ligament using the pad of your thumb. (The falciform ligament lies approximately halfway between the midaxillary line and tip of the xyphoid process along the edge of the rib cage on the right.) Press in a posterior, lateral, and superior direction. Maintain balanced pressure across the falciform ligament with the pad of your thumb until a release occurs and the tension in the ligament dissipates. You will no longer be able to palpate the falciform ligament.

**Figure 10.7** Falciform ligament technique

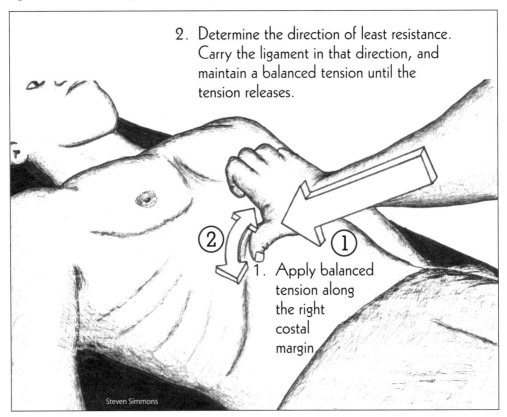

2. Determine the direction of least resistance. Carry the ligament in that direction, and maintain a balanced tension until the tension releases.

② 　 ①

1. Apply balanced tension along the right costal margin

Steven Simmons

## *Superior Linea Alba*

TECHNIQUE: Supine direct myofascial release

SYMPTOMS/DIAGNOSIS: Pain in the epigastric area, indigestion, or shock[4]

PATIENT: Supine

PHYSICIAN: Standing, facing the table at the level of the epigastric area

PROCEDURE: With your hands and fingers perpendicular to the abdomen, line up your fingertips along the linea alba midway between the xyphoid and umbilicus. With straight fingers and hands, and with the fingertips of your index and middle fingers touching their counterparts, press your distal lateral fingertips directly into the midline. Press posteriorly (directly down toward the table) until resistance is met. Maintain steady pressure against this barrier until you feel a release, then rotate the upper portions of your hands closer together and spread your fingertips apart. Once they are fully spread apart, the treatment is complete.

**Figure 10.8** Superior linea alba technique

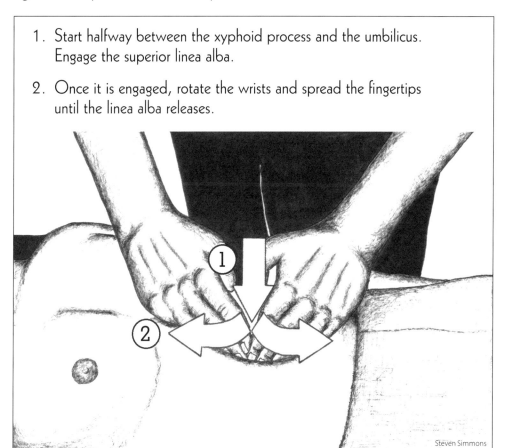

1. Start halfway between the xyphoid process and the umbilicus. Engage the superior linea alba.

2. Once it is engaged, rotate the wrists and spread the fingertips until the linea alba releases.

Steven Simmons

## *Umbilicus*

TECHNIQUE: Supine indirect myofascial release

SYMPTOMS/DIAGNOSIS: Abdominal pain, asthma, pelvic pain, or gastrointestinal complaints

PATIENT: Supine

PHYSICIAN: Standing, facing the table slightly inferior to the umbilicus

PROCEDURE: Inspect the umbilicus for folds along its rim. (A smooth, rounded contour is normal.) Use the pad of your thumb to make contact with the umbilicus. Press deep enough to disengage the umbilicus, then rotate the thumb clockwise and counterclockwise to determine in which direction the umbilicus most easily moves. Rotate steadily in the direction of least resistance until your thumb has turned a full 360°. Stand on the patient's right if you want to go clockwise, and on the patient's left if you want to go counterclockwise. When a barrier is met, maintain steady, balanced pressure against the resistance until a release is felt. Slowly remove your thumb from on top of the umbilicus and inspect to see whether the fold or folds have decreased or disappeared.

**Figure 10.9** Umbilicus technique

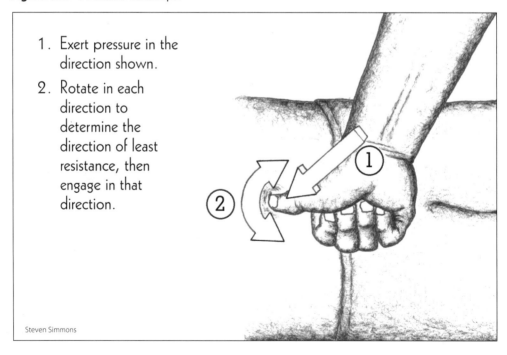

1. Exert pressure in the direction shown.

2. Rotate in each direction to determine the direction of least resistance, then engage in that direction.

Steven Simmons

## *Median Umbilical Ligament*

TECHNIQUE: Supine direct myofascial release

SYMPTOMS/DIAGNOSIS: Pain in suprapubic area or urinary frequency

PATIENT: Supine

PHYSICIAN: Standing, facing the table at the level of the median umbilical ligament

PROCEDURE: With the hands and fingers perpendicular to the abdomen, line up the fingertips along the linea alba halfway between the pubic symphysis and the umbilicus. With flat hands, straight fingers, and the fingertips of the index and middle fingers of each hand touching their counterparts, press the ulnar aspects of the fingertips directly into the midline. Press posteriorly (directly down toward the table) until resistance is met. Maintain steady pressure against this barrier until it begins to melt, then rotate the upper portions of your hands closer together and spread your fingertips apart. Once they are fully spread apart, the treatment is complete.

**Figure 10.10** Median umbilical ligament technique

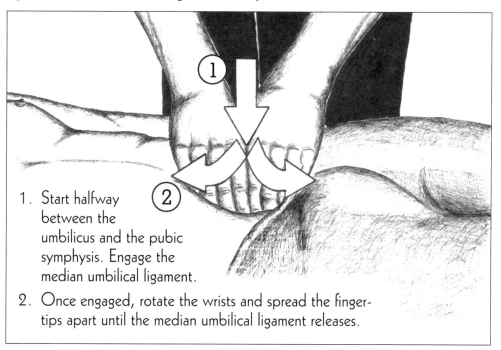

1. Start halfway between the umbilicus and the pubic symphysis. Engage the median umbilical ligament.

2. Once engaged, rotate the wrists and spread the fingertips apart until the median umbilical ligament releases.

## *Presacral Fascia*

TECHNIQUE: Supine direct myofascial release

SYMPTOMS/DIAGNOSIS: Pelvic pain, sacral restriction, low back pain, testicular swelling or hydroceles

PATIENT: Supine

PHYSICIAN: Standing, facing the side of the table at the level of the pelvis

PROCEDURE: The presacral fascia extends down the anterior surface of the sacrum as a continuation of the prevertebral fascia, and attaches to the anterior surface of vertebra S2. You are effecting a change in the presacral fascia by means of the medial umbilical ligaments, which attach to the presacral fascia. You will notice from the effect that this technique has on testicular swelling that you are also affecting strains in the inguinal rings.

Form a horseshoe with your thumb and the middle finger of your dominant hand contacting the medial umbilical ligaments at approximately the level of the deep inguinal rings. These are located about two inches above the pubes and about two inches from the midline. Press posteriorly and slightly inferiorly, maintaining a balanced tension until the release occurs. When it does, you should feel a caudad and cephalad pivoting motion, which follows the internal curve of the sacrum.

**Figure 10.11** Presacral fascia technique

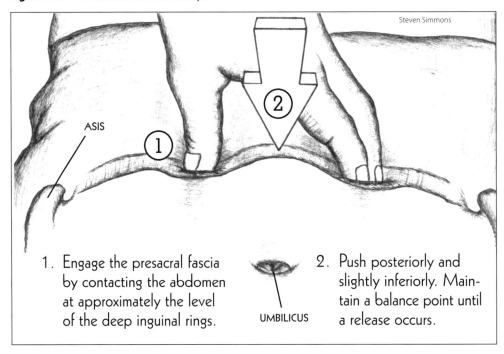

1. Engage the presacral fascia by contacting the abdomen at approximately the level of the deep inguinal rings.

UMBILICUS

2. Push posteriorly and slightly inferiorly. Maintain a balance point until a release occurs.

**Figure 10.12** Presacral fascia technique: lateral view

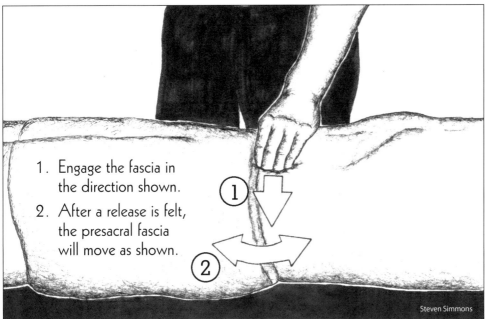

1. Engage the fascia in the direction shown.
2. After a release is felt, the presacral fascia will move as shown.

Steven Simmons

## *Pelvic Diaphragm*

TECHNIQUE: Supine direct myofascial release

SYMPTOMS/DIAGNOSIS: Urinary frequency, pain in the rectum, prostatitis, hemorrhoids, dyspareunia, or pain in the abdomen mimicking left ovarian pain

PATIENT: Supine, with the knees together and flexed to approximately 90° and the feet about a foot apart on the table

PHYSICIAN: Seated on the opposite side to be treated at midthigh level, facing the patient's head

PROCEDURE: Check both sides and then treat the one that is tense, not the one that is lax. Using your right hand to treat the left pelvic diaphragm (or your left hand to treat the right pelvic diaphragm), work on the far side of the pelvis. To engage the diaphragm, follow the natural curve of the medial surface of the far ischial tuberosity, pressing superiorly and laterally with the tip of your thumb. If a firm barrier is met, that layer of the pelvic diaphragm is in spasm. Maintain a steady balanced pressure until a release occurs and that layer softens.

When the outer layer has released, be sure to treat the inner layer by continuing to press in a more superior and lateral direction until a second barrier is felt. Maintain a firm, balanced tension until a second release occurs.

**Figure 10.13** Pelvic diaphragm technique

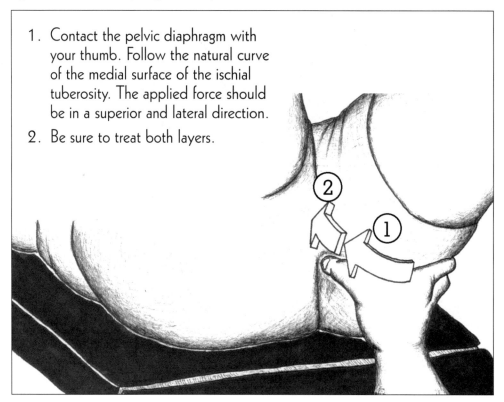

1. Contact the pelvic diaphragm with your thumb. Follow the natural curve of the medial surface of the ischial tuberosity. The applied force should be in a superior and lateral direction.
2. Be sure to treat both layers.

## *Iliotibial Tract*

TECHNIQUE: Supine direct myofascial release

SYMPTOMS/DIAGNOSIS: Pain down the lateral aspect of the thigh

PATIENT: Supine

PHYSICIAN: Standing or seated, facing the affected thigh

PROCEDURE: Locate the tightest point in the tract along the lateral aspect of the thigh. Using the pad of your dominant thumb, reinforced by your other thumb, press medially and posteriorly on this point. Maintain this balanced pressure until a release occurs. The pressure is in the 10- to 30-pound range.

**Figure 10.14**  Iliotibial tract technique

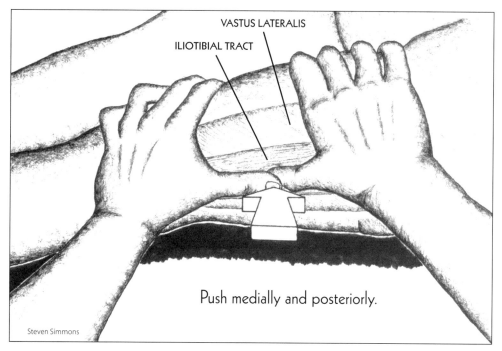

VASTUS LATERALIS

ILIOTIBIAL TRACT

Push medially and posteriorly.

Steven Simmons

## *Fibular Head*

TECHNIQUE: Supine direct ligamentous articular release

SYMPTOMS/DIAGNOSIS: Posterior and lateral knee pain or unstable ankle with chronic spraining of the ankle. The latter is a result of an unstable ankle mortise with the fibula displaced at the knee.

PATIENT: Supine

PHYSICIAN: Seated, facing the side of the table at the level of the affected knee

PROCEDURE: Flex the hip and the knee to approximately 90°. Slightly externally rotate the femur. With the arm closest to the patient's head, bend your elbow to 90° and prop it on the table, making a vertical pedestal with your forearm and thumb. With the pad of this thumb, push the posterior superior portion of the fibular head inferiorly toward the foot. The distal hand inverts the foot and slightly rotates the foot medially. This pulls on the distal end of the fibula. Balance the connective tissue surrounding both ends of the fibula and the interosseous membrane between the tibia and fibula until a release occurs. The fibular head moves inferiorly and anteriorly and slides back into its socket.

**Figure 10.15**  Fibular head technique

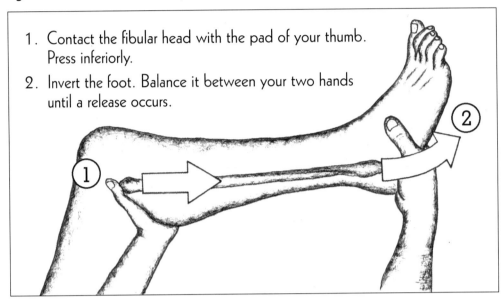

1. Contact the fibular head with the pad of your thumb. Press inferiorly.

2. Invert the foot. Balance it between your two hands until a release occurs.

---

1   Lippincott, H. A., "The Osteopathic Technique of Wm. G. Sutherland, D.O.," 1949 Yearbook of the Academy of Applied Osteopathy, reprint, pp. 19–20

2   Remember that in the embryo, the heart forms above the head and then rotates and moves down through the area of the suprasternal space, dragging all the connective tissue with it. The connective tissue becomes the pericardium, the mediastinum, and central tendon of the diaphragm. As a result, the close inter-relationship between the anterior cervical fascia of the neck and the medi-astinum becomes quite apparent.

3   The use of adjacent tissue to achieve an affect holds true for other techniques as well, for example, the presacral fascia (which uses the medial umbilical ligament and fold).

4   This was one of the main techniques used by Robert Fulford, D.O., to rid the body of the effects of shock, which often inhibit the healing process.

# CHAPTER ELEVEN

# Coordinating the Eight Diaphragms

# Description of the Eight Diaphragms

Osteopathic physicians often find repeated restrictions in certain areas of the body. Sometimes it is the thoracolumbar junction, sometimes the pelvic diaphragm, sometimes the foot, and sometimes other areas. We believe that these common areas of dysfunction act as baffles or dams which prevent the flow of fluid throughout the body. Since the early 1980s members of the Dallas Osteopathic Study Group have identified eight crucial areas of the body that act as diaphragms. These areas augment (when they are functional) or inhibit (when they are dysfunctional) the flow of interstitial fluids.

We cannot overemphasize the importance of this fluid flow. A treatment is finished when the fluids freely "slosh" from end to end, from head to toe. If this does not occur, your treatment will not have a lasting effect, regardless of what else you have done for the patient. When you feel this flow (described below) you do not need to see the patient again for at least a couple weeks. At that point, you determine if any new strains have occurred, or if old areas of compensation have surfaced. You treat the new strains, and when you have everything flowing from one end to the other, the treatment for that session is finished. When the patient enters your office with everything moving with the tide, the patient may be released and told to return only if they reinjure themselves.

To understand the functioning of the diaphragms, one must first understand the flow of the interstitial fluid in the body. Our view is based on Rollin Becker's analogy of the capillary beds acting like a seine lying flat on a beach, washed by the tides of interstitial fluid (see Chapter 3). Based on this analogy, we visualize that the area of dysfunction constitutes a region where the interstitial fluid is not moving. The cells within this area are existing at a lower level of vitality than those in areas with normal interstitial fluid flow.

Once the inhibitions to the flow of interstitial fluid have been removed by correcting the somatic dysfunction, the waste products can be released from the area of restriction where the pain was localized and intense. This also accounts for the temporary spread of *rebound pain* to a broader area. As the "tide" moves back and forth through this area, it washes the waste products into the general circulation of the body where it is carried off by the liver, kidneys, lungs, and skin. This cleansing process is usually completed within eight to thirty-six hours after the correction of the dysfunction. This is when the rebound pain is resolved.

When functioning properly, each of the eight diaphragms augments the movement of the interstitial fluid. When a diaphragm is dysfunctional, it blocks the wave motion of interstitial fluid like a baffle in a gas tank stops the slosh of gasoline.[1]

The endpoint of a treatment session is when all eight diaphragms are working, and the interstitial fluid is felt to be ebbing and flowing from head to toe.

The function of the eight diaphragms is evaluated by feeling for the quality—its volume and smoothness of flow—of the tide flowing through each diaphragm. Pay attention to the amplitude and the quality of the tide rather than its frequency. Remove obstructions to the flow of the interstitial fluid; this allows the tide to move more smoothly and at its optimum amplitude.

During our sixteen years of study with Rollin Becker, members of the study group repeatedly asked him how long each treatment session should last, since it looked like there were a million things to treat. He said, "Just when it's done." But when is it done? He replied:

> When the whole thing's rhythmically going into flexion and extension. That's when your treatment is done for that day. Don't just keep hammering on them, and don't overtreat them. When you've got that going, you don't want to see them again until you have something to work with.[2]

In other words, after you have treated your patient you can tell them, "Okay, we've eliminated some of the strains that your body was not able to free up. You're going to keep working through other dysfunctions that your body can correct until you hit a strain it cannot handle and you plateau. I want to see you at that plateau before I treat you again." When the patient comes into your office for a follow-up visit and their body is working and doing things pretty well, that is, everything is moving (rhythmically going into flexion and extension), they do not need further treatment. You want to have something to treat. You want them "hung up" somewhere before you treat them again.

How do you time your treatments? You estimate how long it is going to be before the patient reaches their next plateau, and this is where experience is valuable. You want to see them within a few days or a couple of weeks after they have hit that plateau so you will have something to treat. When we talk about being "hung up," or at a "plateau," it doesn't mean that the patient has gotten worse, only that they have stopped improving.

Again, it is important not to overtreat. *One of the uses of the eight diaphragms is to let you know when you are through treating a patient for the day.* For the diaphragms to function properly, the surrounding tissues and joints must also be functioning properly. When assessing the status of the flow, start at one end of the body and move to the other end.

The eight diaphragms are:

1. Plantar fascia
2. Knee diaphragm

   a. Popliteal fascia

   b. Cruciate ligaments and transverse ligament of the knee

3. Pelvic diaphragm

4. Respiratory diaphragm

5. Thoracic outlet

   c. Anterior cervical fascia

   d. Subclavius muscles, costocoracoid ligaments and costoclavicular ligaments

6. Suboccipital triangle

7. Tentorium cerebelli

8. Diaphragm sellae

If you find a restriction in one of the eight diaphragms, look for and treat the dysfunctional tissues and/or joints in that area that are inhibiting the diaphragm's function.

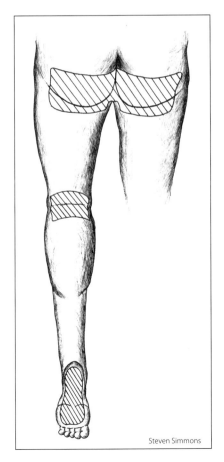

**Figure 11.1** Plantar fascia, popliteal fascia, and pelvic diaphragm

Steven Simmons

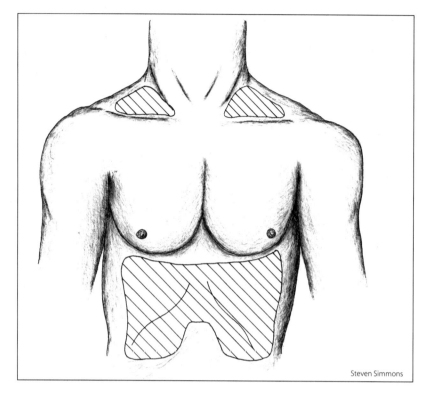

**Figure 11.2**
Respiratory diaphragm and anterior cervical fascia

Steven Simmons

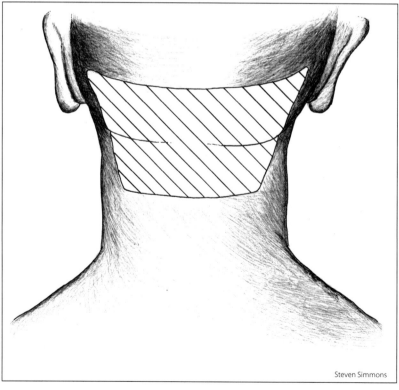

**Figure 11.3**
Suboccipital fascia

Steven Simmons

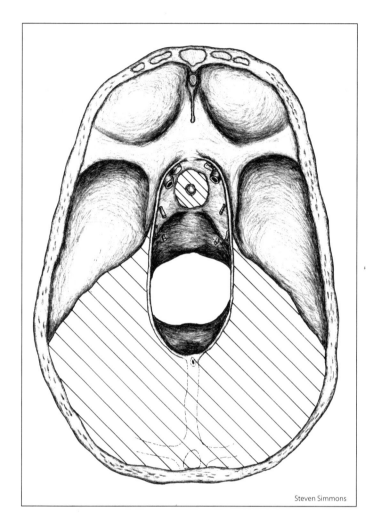

**Figure 11.4**
Tentorirum cerebelli
and diaphragm sellae

Steven Simmons

# Palpating the Diaphragms

Flow in the eight diaphragms is evaluated by feeling the *quality* of the cranial rhythmic impulse. By contrast, merely counting the cranial rhythmic impulse is like counting the pebbles on a beach. It is the quality (vitality, smoothness, and volume) *more than the rate* of that motion that is important. Focus on the quality; for example, liberate a blocked tide and get it moving, or increase the volume of a cranial rhythmic impulse that is moving at a quarter or half of its optimal amplitude. In assessing the quality of the cranial rhythmic impulse or tide, you are feeling for its vitality, smoothness of motion, and amplitude.

Start by checking the plantar fascia, which should be soft so that the cranial rhythmic impulse can flow through it. Once you free up the plantar fascia, move up to the popliteal fossa and release the fascia behind the knee.

Next, check the pelvic diaphragm, remembering that the sacrum is attached to it. Just because you can detect some motion in the sacrum does not mean that the sacrum is fully functional. It is functional when it goes into *full flexion and full extension.*

What if the sacrum is moving but only at a quarter of its full swing? To correct this, check to see if something attached to the sacrum is in dysfunction, since the sacrum cannot swing fully if a tether, the pubococcygeal muscle for example, is in spasm. Once the pelvic diaphragm has been released, what if the cranial rhythmic impulse has increased to only half its optimal amplitude? You should then check the presacral fascia. If releasing the fascia increases the amplitude to only sixty percent, check the iliolumbar ligaments, and release them. Then, lets say it's up to eighty percent. Check and free the occiput off the atlas. Upon rechecking the sacrum you should find it to be one hundred percent functional.

Whether the expected amplitude of the cranial rhythmic impulse is half or quarter of normal, check the presacral fascia, the pelvic diaphragm, the iliolumbar ligaments, etc., releasing each as needed and evaluating the effect they have on the amplitude of the swing of the sacrum. Whatever part of the body you are treating, evaluate the tethers on that area. The Key Lesion is the most important tether, restricting the movement of the entire body.

Next, check for torsion in the pelvis and treat as described in Chapter 5. There are many structures that go through the pelvic diaphragm—rectum, urethra, and vagina—and many people suffer from pelvic diaphragm dysfunctions. Frequent urination is a common problem. Hemorrhoids are also very common. If the pelvic diaphragm is working properly, it is unlikely that a patient would have hemorrhoid problems, since they are varicose veins in a local muscle that is in spasm. Suppose you have loosened the pelvic diaphragm and the presacral fascia and eliminated the torsion in the pelvis. If the sacrum is still not moving correctly, check and release the atlas and occiput since, as we know, the dura connects the occiput to the sacrum. Recheck the sacrum to see if the mechanism is in full swing.

Next is the respiratory diaphragm, which is another area that can act as a baffle. When the respiratory diaphragm acts as a baffle, it prevents the normal up-and-down motion of the fluid. Perhaps more importantly, the respiratory diaphragm may not be *augmenting* that motion. *Each one of these diaphragms, when they are working properly, augments the fluid motion, rather than inhibiting it.*

The treatment of the respiratory diaphragm is described in Chapter 6. Simply, put the heel of your hand in the area of the umbilicus and push the abdominal viscera, primarily the small and large intestines, up into the diaphragm. It is also important to treat the spine in the thoracolumbar region. Now suppose that you are getting better movement in the area, but it is still not quite right. Laterally compress the lower thorax (diaphragm and lower ribs) to further free up those structures. You should then get better movement there.

The respiratory diaphragm has many structures passing through it: the esophagus, abdominal aorta, vena cava, nerves, and lymphatic vessels. Therefore, if you free up the respiratory diaphragm, you augment the return of blood back to the heart as well.

One topic we did not discuss previously was the lymphatic pump. Briefly, it is a technique which involves rhythmic compression or traction of the thorax, respiratory diaphragm, or the feet to augment thoracic excursion and move fluids through the body. This is done to improve venous and lymphatic drainage. Becker's lymphatic pump[3] is as follows:

1. To release the respiratory diaphragm, starting from just above the umbilicus, using the palm of your hand gently scoop up the upper abdominal viscera and compress them up into the lower thorax. If it feels like you have a fully inflated basketball in the palm of your hand, lymphatic fluid is trapped in the abdomen. Gently but firmly compress until the basketball deflates. The fluid has moved across the diaphragm into the thoracic duct. When the "basketball" goes flat, you are done with that part of the treatment.

2. Next, free the sternum as described in Chapter 6 so that the thoracic duct can dump freely into the venous system.

The next diaphragm to be examined is the anterior cervical fascia and the thoracic outlet. The brachial plexus and the venous return from the head and neck pass through this region. Venous congestion in the head often causes headaches. Have you seen people with tortuous veins in their neck? Free up the anterior cervical fascia, and you will often see the pressure go down.

Treating the anterior cervical fascia, because of its relationship with the sympathetic nervous system, is important when treating patients with carpal tunnel syndrome. In addition, treating this diaphragm will help patients with thoracic outlet syndrome or any compression of the brachial plexus.

Last, we have the suboccipital triangle. The vagus nerve exits the skull here, and its impingement can cause many different symptoms since the connections of the vagus nerve are manifold. For example, it goes to the heart, and its impingement can cause idiopathic arrythmias. It continues on into the gut to innervate the stomach and part of the bowels. When the parasympathetic flow is decreased there is usually a relative increase in sympathetic flow. An increase in sympathetic activity in the stomach decreases the mucosal barrier of the stomach lining, leading to stomach ulcers, and colic in infants.

Then move to the head and check the tentorium cerebelli and the diaphragm sellae. The importance of treating these diaphragms cannot be overemphasized, and are well described in texts on cranial osteopathy.[4]

# Techniques for Treating the Eight Diaphragms

## Plantar Fascia

TECHNIQUE: Supine direct myofascial release

SYMPTOMS/DIAGNOSIS: Pain on the bottom of the foot, heel spurs, or plantar fasciitis

PATIENT: Supine

PHYSICIAN: Seated at the foot of the table

PROCEDURE: Your thumbs are crossed and the pads are pressed into the plantar fascia at the level of the tarsal-metatarsal junctions, with your fingers

**Figure 11.5** Plantar fascia technique

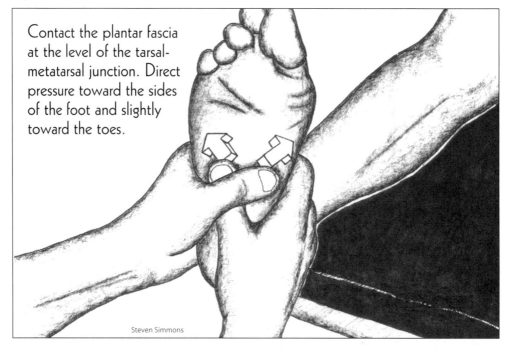

Contact the plantar fascia at the level of the tarsal-metatarsal junction. Direct pressure toward the sides of the foot and slightly toward the toes.

Steven Simmons

interlaced across the dorsum of the foot. The pads of the thumbs press in the direction the thumbs are pointed, that is, toward either side of the foot and slightly toward the toes, and are taken to a point of balanced tension. Once a release occurs, the tips of your thumbs seem to slip across the fascia. Repeat the same procedure with the toes in plantar flexion. Once that release occurs, repeat the procedure with the toes in dorsiflexion. The treatment of the plantar fascia is complete once you have accomplished all three releases.

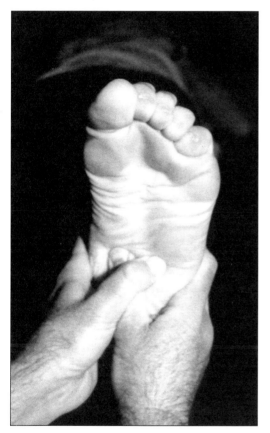

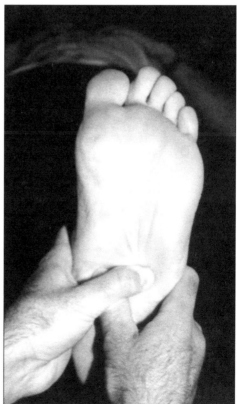

**Figure 11.6** Plantar flexion

Instruct the patient to "step on the gas," forcing the foot into plantar flexion.

**Figure 11.7** Dorsiflexion

Instruct the patient to bend the toes toward the head.

## *Popliteal Fascia*

TECHNIQUE Supine direct myofascial release

SYMPTOMS/DIAGNOSIS: Pain behind the knee or Baker's cyst

PATIENT: Supine

PHYSICIAN: Seated at the side of the table inferior to the patient's knee, facing the head of the table

PROCEDURE: With the patient's leg relaxed, place your fingertips just above the popliteal fossa. The fingers of both hands are bent with the lateral fingernails of your little fingers and ring fingers touching and the heels of your hands approximately three inches apart. The fingers will form a plough- or wedge-like shape. Grasp the tissue under your hands and draw them inferiorly toward the foot. If resistance is met, maintain balanced tension inferiorly and anteriorly until this barrier "melts" and your fingers slide inferiorly, with the popliteal fascia melting ahead of the little fingers.

**Figure 11.8** Popliteal fascia technique

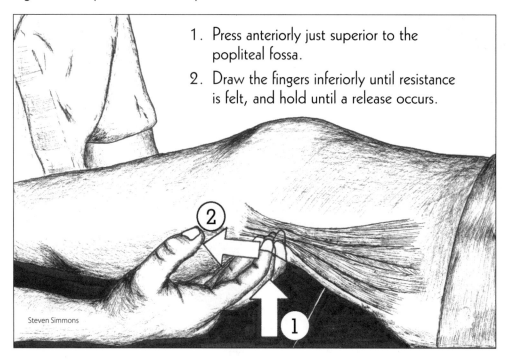

1. Press anteriorly just superior to the popliteal fossa.
2. Draw the fingers inferiorly until resistance is felt, and hold until a release occurs.

Steven Simmons

# Pelvic Diaphragm

The muscles and organs of the pelvic cavity connect with the endopelvic fascia. The endopelvic fascia in turn is connected to the medial umbilical ligaments, which connect to the umbilicus and the linea alba of the rectus sheath. Continuing superiorly from the umbilicus, the falciform ligaments and the round ligament of the liver, that is, the remnant of umbilical vein, attach to the liver as well as to the inferior surface of the diaphragm. Therefore, there is a direct anterior connection from the pelvic diaphragm to the respiratory diaphragm. The falciform ligament, round ligament, and the venous ligament run anterior to posterior and basically divide the liver into lobes. Thus, not only is there an inferior to superior connection from the pelvic diaphragm to the respiratory diaphragm, there is also an anterior to posterior connection of the anterior abdominal wall and posterior wall under the diaphragm. For the discussion here, it is important to note that:

1. The pelvic diaphragm is made up of two separate fascial planes.

2. The pelvic diaphragm acts like a diaphragm by pumping fluids from the lower extremities into the abdominal cavity.

TECHNIQUE: Supine direct myofascial release

SYMPTOMS/DIAGNOSIS: Urinary frequency, pain in the rectum, prostatitis, hemorrhoids, dyspareunia, or pain in the abdomen mimicking left ovarian pain

PATIENT: Supine, with the knees together and flexed to approximately 90º and the feet about a foot apart on the table

PHYSICIAN: Seated on the opposite side to be treated at midthigh level, facing the patient's head

PROCEDURE: Check both sides and then treat the one that is tense, not the one that is lax. Using your right hand to treat the left pelvic diaphragm (or left hand to treat the right pelvic diaphragm), work on the far side of the pelvis. To engage the diaphragm, follow the natural curve of the medial surface of the far ischial tuberosity, pressing superiorly and laterally with the tip of your thumb. If a firm barrier is met, that layer of the pelvic diaphragm is in spasm. Maintain a steady balanced pressure until a release occurs and that layer softens.

When the outer layer has released, be sure to treat the inner layer by continuing to press in a more superior and lateral direction until a second barrier is felt. Maintain a firm balanced tension until a second release occurs.

In our experience, the left pelvic diaphragm appears to be more dysfunctional than the right. Also note that if both sides are tight, treating the tighter side often releases the other side.

**Figure 11.9** Pelvic diaphragm technique

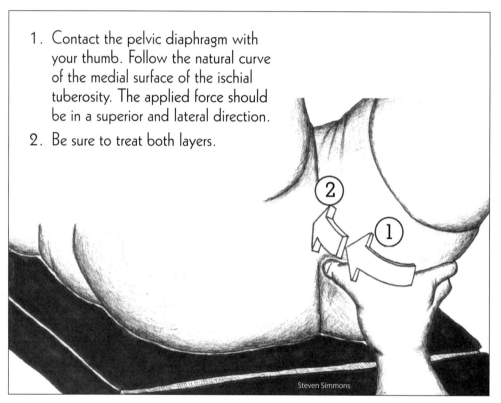

1. Contact the pelvic diaphragm with your thumb. Follow the natural curve of the medial surface of the ischial tuberosity. The applied force should be in a superior and lateral direction.
2. Be sure to treat both layers.

Steven Simmons

## *Respiratory Diaphragm*

TECHNIQUE: Supine direct myofascial release

SYMPTOMS/DIAGNOSIS: Inability to take a deep breath

PATIENT: Supine

PHYSICIAN: Standing at the side of the table, facing the patient's head at approximately the level of the pelvis

PROCEDURE: Using the heel of your dominant hand, scoop up the viscera, starting from just above the umbilicus. Be careful not to traumatize the aorta. Compress the viscera in a superior direction toward the lower chest, causing the upper portion of the respiratory diaphragm to rise to form a smooth dome. Remember that the diaphragm acts like a piston, and occasionally the piston gets stuck in a downward position. Maintain firm, balanced pressure until the respiratory diaphragm relaxes. This procedure also moves any lymphatic fluid trapped below the diaphragm in the cisterna chyli up across the diaphragm and into the thoracic duct.

Also, if needed, you can treat the midthoracic spine at the same time by grasping across the thoracic paravertebral muscles in the area of the dysfunction with your nondominant hand, and maintaining pressure between your two hands. If this is done, the procedure is complete when you feel the thoracic dysfunction relax in your nondominant hand, and the "balloon" collapse in the palm of your dominant hand.

**Figure 11.10**  Respiratory diaphragm technique

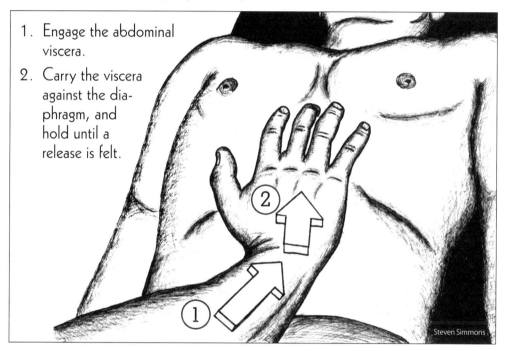

1. Engage the abdominal viscera.
2. Carry the viscera against the diaphragm, and hold until a release is felt.

Steven Simmons

## *Anterior Cervical Fascia*

TECHNIQUE: Supine direct myofascial release

SYMPTOMS/DIAGNOSIS: Globus hystericus, headache, pain or numbness in the arm or hand on the affected side, pain medial to shoulder blade on the affected side, tightness in the supraclavicular fossae

PATIENT: Supine

PHYSICIAN: Seated at the head of the table, facing the patient's feet

PROCEDURE: Place the pads of your thumbs in the supraclavicular fossa on either side of the sternal notch, just lateral to the sternocleidomastoid muscles. Press your thumbs inferiorly, straight toward the patient's feet. Treat the tight side with balanced pressure. Your other thumb may be removed. (Both sides may be tight; in that case, both sides can be treated at the same time.) Once the tightness in the tissue under your thumb(s) dissipates, draw the pads of your thumbs laterally toward the acromioclavicular joints. The tight fascia and anterior scalene muscles will melt ahead of your thumb. This area is very sensitive, so take great care to use the precise amount of balanced pressure necessary to achieve the release. If you let the patient know that you are aware of this tenderness, he or she can better tolerate the discomfort until the release occurs.

It should be noted that:

1. Releasing the anterior cervical fascia will result in a release of the anterior scalene and the omohyoid muscles.

2. Always press directly with the pads of your thumbs. In this case, they are parallel to the clavicles and pointed toward the sternoclavicular joint. Avoid pushing your thumbs sideways, as this would sprain the distal joints of the thumbs.

**Figure 11.11** Anterior cervical fascia technique

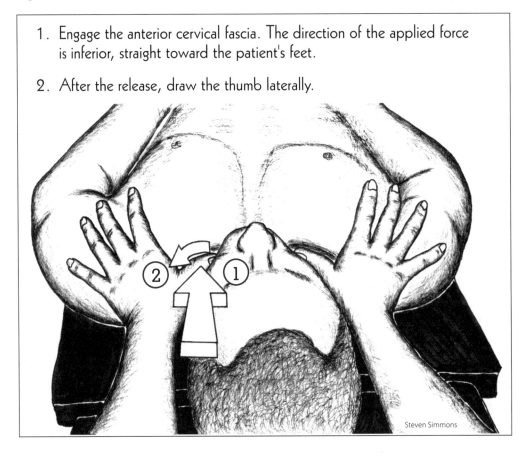

1. Engage the anterior cervical fascia. The direction of the applied force is inferior, straight toward the patient's feet.

2. After the release, draw the thumb laterally.

Steven Simmons

# Suboccipital Fascia

SYMPTOMS/DIAGNOSIS: Neck pain and/or cephalagia

PATIENT: Supine, approximately 8 inches down from the head of the table

PHYSICIAN: Sitting at the head of the table

PROCEDURE: Place the thenar eminences of your supine hands under either side of the back of the head along the tentorium, with the fingertips on the atlas. The fingertips are carried anteriorly and superiorly toward the patient's eyes until the atlas glides forward on the occipital condyles. Maintain balanced tension between the tentorium and the area of dysfunction until a release occurs.

**Figure 11.12**  Suboccipital fascia hand position

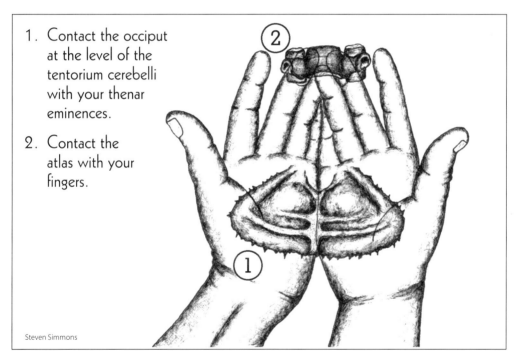

1. Contact the occiput at the level of the tentorium cerebelli with your thenar eminences.

2. Contact the atlas with your fingers.

Steven Simmons

# Tentorium Cerebelli and Diaphragm Sellae

The treatment of these areas should be done with one of the many techniques of cranial osteopathy. Osteopathy in the cranial field has been very well described by Harold I. Magoun and will not be covered in this text.[5]

1   A baffle in a gas tank keeps the fluid from sloshing. That works well for a gas tank, but we want the fluids to slosh around in the body. So if they are working like baffles, we are going to try and help them turn back into diaphragms. You want everything working together, and everything moving.

2   Comment of Rollin Becker at a monthly meeting of the Dallas Osteopathic Study Group.

3   Ibid.

4   Sutherland WG. *Teachings in the Science of Osteopathy*, ed. Anne L. Wales. Portland, OR: Rudra Press, 1990: 187.

5   Magoun HI. *Osteopathy in the Cranial Field*, 3rd ed. Indianapolis, IN: The Cranial Academy, 1976: 25.

# CONCLUSION

Just as we at the Dallas Osteopathic Study Group have stood on the shoulders of our mentors and predecessors to improve our view of Osteopathy, so too is this book intended to provide the reader with another small shoulder on which to stand. We hope that it will provide future generations of Osteopathic Physicians with another step up to the basic truths in nature.

The value of study groups cannot be overemphasized. Dr. William Sutherland taught his techniques through a study group. Dr. Rollin Becker continued this tradition by establishing the Dallas Osteopathic Study Group in 1963 to further the goals of Osteopathy. Study groups provide an open-minded environment for individuals to freely express their creativity and to bounce ideas off their peers. Whole new techniques and concepts can thereby be developed. The result is the advancement of each participant's skills and the improvement of techniques to relieve human suffering.

# INDEX